STROKE:
The Road to Recovery
A Guide for Survivors & Families

Dr. F. Douglas Prillaman, Ed.D.
and
Tom Willett

Introduction and medical commentary by noted neurologist
Dr. S. James Shafer, M.D.

Alva Pyddison

STROKE

ISBN-13: 978-0615830278
ISBN-10: 0615830277

The information presented in this book or its associated websites and social media pages is offered for informational purposes only. Nothing herein should be construed as the giving of advice or the making of a recommendation regarding any decision or action related to your health or the health of others.

This information is not meant to be used, nor should it be used, to diagnose or treat any medical condition. Nor should it be used as a substitute for consultation with practicing medical professionals. For diagnosis or treatment of any medical problem, consult your physician.

While the authors and publisher have used reasonable efforts to ensure that the information herein is accurate, complete and current, we expressly disclaim any warranty or representation regarding the accuracy, completeness or currency of such information. This information is provided "As Is," without warranty of any kind, express or implied.

For Eleanor

Words cannot express the deep debt of gratitude
I owe you for sacrificing your life for mine.

...

CONTENTS

Prologue   1

Introduction   5

Chapter 1   You've Had a Stroke   7

Chapter 2   Causes of Stroke & Its Diagnosis   15
             Dr. S. James Shafer, M.D.

Chapter 3   Effects of Stroke   23

Chapter 4   Early Treatment of Stroke   29

Chapter 5   Admission to the Rehab Hospital   37

Chapter 6   Life as a Long-Term Inpatient   41

Chapter 7   Current Practices in Treatment   45
             of Stroke
             Dr. S. James Shafer, M.D.

Chapter 8   Early Attempts at Rehabilitation   53

Chapter 9   The Role of the Physical Therapist   57

Chapter 10   The Role of the Occupational   65
             Therapist

Chapter 11   The Role of the Speech Therapist   69

Chapter 12   The Roles of the Psychological &   73
             Recreational Therapists

Chapter 13   Two Steps Forward, One Step Back   77

Chapter 14   Making the House More Accessible   81

Chapter 15   Outpatient Therapy & Home   89
             Health Care

Chapter 16	Public Accessibility	93
Chapter 17	Caregiving *A Word from Eleanor Prillaman*	99
Chapter 18	Continued Therapies at Home	117
Chapter 19	Coping with Pain	129
Chapter 20	Dealing with Depression	133
Chapter 21	Closing the Gap Between Theory & Experience	137
Epilogue		141
Postscript		143
Bonus	Understanding Stroke: An *Experiential* Guide to Medical Terminology	145
Bonus	Understanding Stroke: An *Alphabetical* Guide to Medical Terminology	163
Bonus	Stroke Resources	181
Authors		189

www.strokebookonline.com

PROLOGUE

Our hope is that this book will help stroke patients and their families better understand the nature of their illness and the steps toward recovery. Herein we will offer a first-person, plain-English account of one person's stroke, accompanied by medical information on current diagnosis and treatment from an expert in the field of neurology. We've also included an extensive glossary and a list of online resources.

First, a bit about how this book came to be written. After suffering a serious stroke, and spending more than three months as an inpatient at a local rehabilitation hospital, the day I was released felt like Christmas and my birthday all rolled into one. I had never been so happy to leave a place in my life! Between the rigorous schedule of therapy, and the constant struggle with pain and depression, I felt someone had just given me the ultimate "Get Out of Jail Free" card! I had no idea, of course, how many challenges still lay ahead, nor did I want to think about it. I simply wanted to get out of there and get back to my home, my wife and my dog!

My "vacation" from dealing with the stroke was short-lived. On the second day at home, while I was practicing learning to walk again with my son, Tom, he said, "Dad, you ought to write a book about your experiences with the stroke." He seemed to think that since my career, prior to retirement, had involved working with handicapped and disabled children and adults, I might be able to describe what it's like from a certain unique perspective. As he pressed me about it he said, "Think about it! How many people have both the technical knowledge you do about disability, and real first-hand experience? You might really be able to help future stroke survivors."

I believe my first response was, "Damn you!" How could he think I would want to dwell on such a painful and unhappy period of my life, much less write about it? "No," I told him, "I simply can't deal with that part of my life at this time. It will be too painful to relive the past, and I've got to stay focused on moving ahead."

Midst all of my denials, I was reminded that two of my therapists at the rehab hospital, who had endured my running commentary on how I thought they should change the therapeutic process, had already recommended that I put some of my observations in writing—both the good and the bad. At that time I thought about it for a minute, but, having co-authored a textbook[1] during the time I was a professor of Special Education, I didn't look forward to again having to deal with the deadlines, the re-writes, and the search for a publisher. Been there. Done that. But as I continued to mull it over, I slowly began to get excited. "Why not?" I finally concluded. "If I can get a few things off my chest, and perhaps help someone else, I should at least try." Tom and I talked some more, and a few short weeks later we had a working outline.

Knowing how to conclude a book like this is almost as hard as knowing how to start. I by no means consider myself finished with my own recuperation, yet I hope that what follows will help you and your loved ones either prepare for the possibility of a stroke, or begin to find your own way to recovery on the road ahead.

Doug Prillaman
North Hutchinson Island, Florida

---

[1] *Educational Diagnosis and Prescriptive Teaching: A Practical Approach to Special Education in the Least Restrictive Environment;* Douglas Prillaman and John C. Abbott; Fearon Education, Pitman Learning; Belmont, CA © 1983.

Editor's Note: Definitions of words in **bold** can be found in the glossaries beginning on page 145.

INTRODUCTION

Stroke is the fourth leading cause of death in the United States. It is the leading cause of morbidity and disability in both men and women over the age of 60. Multiple mechanisms are responsible for stroke symptoms. In addition, there are numerous causative factors which place certain individuals at increased risk of having a cerebral vascular accident (stroke).

Current understanding regarding the physiology of cerebral vascular disease has enabled physicians to more aggressively treat, and in many instances reverse, the neurological deficits that are experienced with such an event. Unfortunately, tens of thousands of people are still left with severe disabilities because of this crippling disease. Further medical knowledge and, just as importantly, an improved understanding of the immense psychological toll that stroke takes on its victims and their families, is still needed.

The book you are about to read is both a courageous and noble effort by a patient who has suffered the consequences of stroke. In providing the reader with a basic knowledge of the mechanisms and causes of stroke, as well as relating the human side to this trauma, it is hoped that there will be a heightened awareness of the need for continued research into the treatment of stroke and an improved social understanding of this disease process.

Additionally, this book is for those patients who have survived a stroke. We hope that here you may find strength, courage and better understanding, and the realization that you are not alone in what you have experienced.

Dr. S. James Shafer, M.D.
Vero Neurology
Vero Beach, Florida

Chapter 1
YOU'VE HAD A STROKE

My full name is Floyd Douglas Prillaman, but my friends and family call me Doug. I'm a native Virginian, seventy-two years of age and holding.

For the sake of brevity, I'll start my story in 1959 when I was a teacher, counselor and basketball coach at a junior high school in the Tidewater, Virginia area. One night at a P.T.A. meeting I noticed a very attractive blonde as she walked across the stage to give a presentation. I immediately inquired about her and learned that she was a fellow teacher, and a widow with two children. Time flies when you're having fun, and a short six months later we were married. Along with the marriage came an instant family which included not only a daughter, Nancy, and a son, Tom, but Mittens, the cat. Neither of us ever had any respect for one another—the cat and I, that is.

While teaching at the junior high, I had my first encounter with special students—both handicapped and gifted. I found it exciting and challenging, and soon decided I wanted to pursue a career in Special Education. There was much I needed to learn, so I enrolled in graduate courses at the University of Virginia and the College of

William & Mary. After receiving my Masters degree from William & Mary, I returned to the classroom where, as is often the case, my most valuable education came not from formal course work but from the kids and teenagers I taught, and from their parents.

In 1964, I accepted an offer to become the Director of Special Education services for the Arlington County public school system in Virginia. Arlington had a highly-regarded program for all handicapped populations, as well as for the gifted and talented. I worked with and supervised teachers and therapists for five years, gaining much experience while continuing my graduate studies.

Shortly after completing my Doctorate at George Washington University in Washington, DC, I was invited to join the faculty of the College of William & Mary in Williamsburg, Virginia as a Professor of Special Education. In my classes, I trained teachers and school administrators to work with handicapped students. It was during my tenure there that I developed a new approach to Special Ed called the Diagnostic Prescriptive Teacher program. The focus was on trying to eliminate unnecessary labeling of students, and I was eager to implement the program at my alma mater. I had felt for some time that the concept of de-emphasizing labels was both a personal and political issue that needed to be addressed. Naturally enough I met with some resistance, primarily because most of us resist change. After all, "we've done it this way for forty years!" But I hung in there, and in addition to my teaching responsibilities I stayed busy writing grants in order to raise tuition money for teachers who wanted to promote change in the Special

Education services delivery system. Initially, I began to see a change in the thinking of prospective teachers, and finally even some of the decision makers and administrators responded positively. The combination of working directly with students while trying to "change the system" was very gratifying—not a bad way to spend your time if you have to work for a living.

I could have continued on at William & Mary for many years, but in 1992 when the Governor of Virginia announced a plan for early retirement, I decided to opt for the "early out." It was a difficult choice, but I felt confident that my training and experiences were such that I could return to a similar position at a later date if I chose to do so.

The simplest way I know to describe a stroke is that if the brain is deprived of the oxygen and nutrients it normally gets from blood, and if the lack of blood goes on long enough, the cells in the effected area can die.

Early retirement provided many options for me and my family. Preferring the beach and warmer climes (a predilection I developed while on loan to The College of the Virgin Islands in St. Thomas), my wife and I sold our rambling home in Williamsburg and moved to an oceanfront condominium on the Treasure Coast of Florida. From time to time I thought about part-time teaching if some college needed an adjunct professor, but mostly I spent my time reading, cooking, bread-making and studying to be a beach bum.

The Day of the Stroke

The good life agreed with us. We developed many new friendships and kept up a lively, though relaxed, pace of dining out and traveling. I was even having my first real success at quitting smoking—a habit I had enjoyed since my teens. The drug I was taking to reduce my craving for nicotine really worked, but it had some nasty side effects including dizziness and nausea. In hope of finding some relief, we scheduled an appointment with my doctor.

It was a typical Florida afternoon, with a brief thunder-storm making our drive across town to the doctor's office both stressful and tiresome. We parked the car, and when I got out, without warning my legs crumpled and I hit the pavement! I got up quickly, brushed myself off and insisted to my wife that I was all right. Once inside, the doctor gave me a brief checkup and decided that it was just the dizziness that I had been experiencing from the medication. We agreed that if I wanted to continue on with the drug, I would just have to put up with the side effects.

We drove home, somewhat relieved, yet, as I got out of the car in the parking lot of our condominium, I fell again! This time we had to have several neighbors help me up. With a borrowed wheelchair, and growing concern, we made it back into our condo.

All I could think of was that I wanted to go lie down. Yet as I got out of the wheelchair, I fell a third time! This time

I couldn't get back to my feet—in fact I couldn't even crawl! Once again, neighbors came to my rescue, and after they got me into bed, my wife announced that she was going to call 911. I begged her not to, because I was sure that it was nothing serious. Yes, one of my outstanding characteristics is my stubbornness. But I didn't want to go to the hospital, and I certainly didn't want to go through the embarrassment of being carried out of my own house on a stretcher and put in an ambulance. We negotiated a compromise, and one of the neighbors drove me to the emergency room, while Eleanor followed in our Jeep.

In the Emergency Room
I must confess that I have only the vaguest memories about what took place over the next several days. I'm sure that's due in part to the shock that one goes through during any major medical incident. Based on subsequent conversations with my doctors and family, plus ongoing reading, I've been able to piece together the following.

When we arrived at the hospital we had to go through the usual "hurry up and wait" process. The **triage nurse** notified the emergency room staff that a patient needed priority attention. Unfortunately, there were several "priority" patients that night, and as I lay on a gurney for the next forty-five minutes it seemed like an eternity. When the doctor on duty finally got to me, he took a medical history while doing a physical exam, and then performed several "bedside neurological tests." During the history, he seemed to be interested in whether I smoked ("yes"), had high blood pressure ("no"), and what medications I was currently taking. The physical included the usual temperature, blood pressure and pulse, plus requests for me to perform various tasks that might provide him clues as to the state of my motor, sensory, language and memory systems. The neurological exam consisted of several standard questions which everyone I met for the next several days seemed to be interested in. "Do you know where you are?" ("The hospital.") "How old are you?" ("Who wants to know?") "Who is the President of the United States?" ("Bill Clinton, and he doesn't know how to keep his pants zipped.") They never seemed to tire of asking the same questions, and I never tired of giving the same answers.

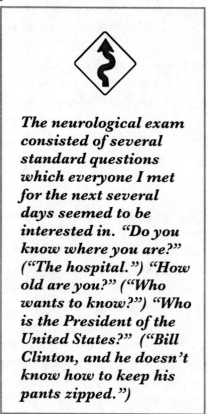

The neurological exam consisted of several standard questions which everyone I met for the next several days seemed to be interested in. "Do you know where you are?" ("The hospital.") "How old are you?" ("Who wants to know?") "Who is the President of the United States?" ("Bill Clinton, and he doesn't know how to keep his pants zipped.")

At this point the doctor announced a preliminary diagnosis that I had suffered a **stroke,** and ordered a series of lab tests. A **cat scan,** a sort of X-ray of the brain, was used to determine if there had been a hemorrhage or some kind of blockage in a major blood vessel. An **MRI** provided even more detailed information by using a large magnetic field and radio waves to create a 3-D picture of my brain. (How I was able to lie still for the forty-five minutes it takes to do the test, I'll never know.) There's also an **MRA** that can take pictures of the veins and arteries, and sometimes they use **Ultrasound.**

Based on what these tests revealed about the condition of my brain, heart and vascular system, we were told that I definitely had an **"infarct"** (the first of many medical terms that had absolutely no meaning to us until we pressed for an explanation). We found out that an infarct is an area of brain tissue that is dead or dying because of loss of blood supply, and with that determination it was clear that I would be formally admitted to the hospital.

Admission to the Hospital

The official time of my admittal was 2:00 a.m., and as luck would have it, my regular doctor, who I had just seen the day before, had left for vacation. Thankfully, out of concern for my dizziness and the first fall, we had asked him for the name of a good **neurologist.** My wife was able to remember the physician he recommended, and Dr. James Shafer was kind enough to take our call in the dead of night and admit me under his care.

For the next nine days I lay in that hospital—five days in **critical care** and four in **progressive care.** My neurologist and the hospital staff focused their energies on stopping the stroke from either progressing or recurring, determining the exact location and extent of damage, and preventing complications from setting in. I was hooked up to all manner of machines, tubes, monitors and alarms.

There were battery after battery of tests designed to observe my heart rate, breathing and brain functions. All I and my family wanted to know was: What happened to me? How bad is it? When will I get better? Unfortunately, with stroke, getting answers to those questions can take several days, and knowing exactly how much physical and mental recovery you will make can take months, even years.

Over the course of my hospital stay, my family and I got a brief education in the science of the brain. The simplest way I know to describe a stroke is that if the brain is deprived of the oxygen and nutrients it normally gets from blood, and if the lack of blood goes on long enough, the cells in the effected area can die. Your blood is being pumped from your heart to your brain via four main passageways: two large arteries on either side of your neck (the **carotid arteries**), and two more that run up your spinal cord (the **vertebral arteries**). The stoppage of blood flow can be caused by a blood vessel either bursting (a **hemorrhage**) or becoming clogged by a blood clot or other particle (an **ischemia**), which is what happened in my case. Further, our brains are basically divided right down the middle into two halves (or hemispheres)—right and left. And within each of these halves there are four main areas that control different mental and physical functions. How a stroke affects you is based in large part on which of these areas is damaged by the lack of blood. I'll leave the rest of the medical terminology to Dr. Shafer, but basically the doctors have to figure out what type of stroke you had and where it occurred before they can determine the proper course of treatment.

Chapter 2
CAUSES OF STROKE & ITS DIAGNOSIS
Dr. S. James Shafer, M.D.

Stroke is the fourth leading cause of death and the most common cause of disability among the elderly within the United States. As such, it is a major health concern and a significant amount of research and resources go into its treatment and prevention. More than 795,000 strokes occur every year in the U.S., resulting in approximately 137,000 deaths per year. In addition to the personal impact on victims and their families, the economic impact of stroke and stroke **rehabilitation** is enormous, and the cost will continue to rise as our population ages and the incidence of stroke increases.

Stroke is the fourth leading cause of death and the most common cause of disability among the elderly within the United States. More than 795,000 strokes occur every year in the U.S., resulting in approximately 137,000 deaths per year.

A stroke, more formally known as a **cerebrovascular** accident or **CVA,** is an event which occurs due to a lack of oxygen to a particular part of the brain, resulting in permanent neurological deficits. Patients who experience stroke may have various neurological symptoms, including **paralysis,** sensory loss, language disturbance and visual field loss.

A basic understanding of the anatomy of the central nervous system will help explain the origin of these symptoms. The brain is divided into right and left halves, or hemispheres. Both hemispheres control motor function for the opposite side of the body. Thus, a person with a right hemispheric stroke may have left-sided paralysis and vice versa. Sensory function is also effected on the opposite side to the hemisphere which is injured.

The **right hemisphere** plays a predominant role in orientation to our environment. Patients who have right hemispheric stroke may experience a phenomenon known as **"neglect"** in which they are unaware of their paralysis and neglect the functions of the left side of their body. They have a tendency to orient to the right side and not recognize stimuli in their left hemibody space.

The **left hemisphere** plays a major role in language function, a complex activity requiring multiple association systems. Some stroke patients are able to understand what is being said to them but have difficulty expressing themselves. They have difficulty producing words and yet may be able to communicate in other fashions such as writing or using sign language. This is known as a "nonfluent" or **"Broca's" aphasia.** Other patients are unable to understand language, have difficulty following commands and commonly produce nonsensical language. This is called "fluent" or **"Wernicke's" aphasia.** The patient with Wernicke's aphasia may appear confused, may not answer questions appropriately and may ramble sentences, producing a "word salad."

The right and left hemispheres work together in bringing meaning association to many stimuli in our environment. Additionally, both hemispheres work together in certain functions of memory.

Further, the brain is divided into areas of subcortical and cortical function. The subcortical regions of the brain contain motor and sensory pathways which connect various parts of the central nervous system to one another. Cortical function occurs in the more advanced portion of the brain known as the gray matter. It is this area which provides association and meaning to virtually all of our sensory and motor systems.

The **cerebellum** or "hind brain" is responsible for the orchestration of limb motor skills and walking (gait) stability. Stroke to this region of the central nervous system results in a lack of coordination of fine motor skills and disorders of gait.

The **brain stem,** which connects the two cerebral hemispheres to the spinal cord, contains three regions known as the midbrain, pons and medulla. The brain stem is the central conduit through which all pathways from the hemispheres travel and connect to the spinal cord, ultimately providing input to the extremities. The brain stem is a compact area of anatomy and even small areas of injury generally result in profound neurological deficits.

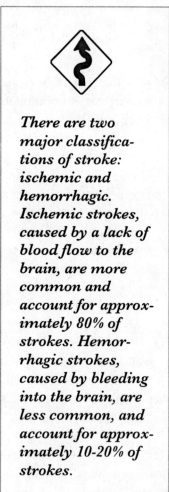

There are two major classifications of stroke: ischemic and hemorrhagic. Ischemic strokes, caused by a lack of blood flow to the brain, are more common and account for approximately 80% of strokes. Hemorrhagic strokes, caused by bleeding into the brain, are less common, and account for approximately 10-20% of strokes.

The blood that flows to each part of the brain carries the oxygen necessary for the brain's function. The nerve cells (or neurons) of the brain can only withstand a few minutes without oxygen before they begin to die. Once stroke occurs, the area of the brain normally fed by the blocked **artery** will suffer neuronal cell death and irreversible damage. Outside of this area is the penumbra (or umbrella), that adjacent portion of the brain which is highly susceptible to further lack of blood flow but remains functioning due to complex compensatory mechanisms. It is upon this surrounding area of brain tissue that post-stroke care focuses its efforts, as not protecting this region can significantly increase stroke-related morbidity.

There are two major classifications of stroke: **ischemic** and **hemorrhagic.** Ischemic strokes are more common and account for approximately 80% of strokes. Ischemic strokes are caused by a lack of blood flow to the brain. The blockage of blood may be caused by either a localized blood clot (a **thrombus**) or by a blood clot that travels through the cardiovascular system (an **embolus**). An embolus can originate in one artery and move to another, or it may come from another source such as the heart. When smaller blood vessels are closed off, the result is often a "subcortical infarction" or "lacunar stroke." This process is most common in patients with atherosclerosis (hardening of the arteries), diabetes and hypertension.

Hemorrhagic strokes are the least common of the two and account for approximately 10-20% of strokes. The name implies that there has been a hemorrhage or bleeding into the brain, often resulting from a ruptured blood vessel. Uncontrolled hypertension is the most common cause of this sort of intracranial hemorrhage.

There are two other kinds of strokes that may occur. An acute onset of neurological deficit which clears up within twenty-four hours is known as a **transient ischemic attack (TIA).** TIA can be a warning sign before a major stroke. TIAs are typically few in number and generally occur in duration of at least ten minutes. Many people refer to them as "mini strokes." Neurological deficits which last longer than twenty-four hours but less than one week are commonly referred to as a reversible ischemic neurological deficit (RIND).

Multiple mechanisms are responsible for stroke. Blood clots that form in the heart and then move to the brain are a common source of stroke. When the upper portion (or atrium) of the heart is in fibrillation (a rapid twitching), blood flow is erratic and a blood clot (a thrombus) may form within the atrial chamber. Portions of this thrombus may break off and pass through the heart, up the aorta and into the carotid or basilar artery systems, the two main passageways which deliver blood to the brain. A blood clot which has started out in a larger blood vessel will sooner or later lodge itself in a smaller vessel, therefore blocking all blood flow beyond the clot. Other sources of cardiac embolism are heart attack (acute myocardial infarction) and heart wall (septal) defects between chambers of the heart.

A further source of stroke may be an event called "artery to artery **thromboembolism,"** when a thrombus (blood clot) travels from one artery to another. The most commonly known source of artery to artery thrombus is carotid artery **stenosis** (narrowing). The carotid arteries are the two main blood vessels which feed the anterior (or forward) part of the brain. Arteries over time may experience narrowing as a consequence of atherosclerosis. The areas of atherosclerosis become sources of thrombus formation. If a thrombus continues to form within these atherosclerotic plaques, then eventually they may dislodge and travel into the brain, blocking an artery and causing stroke symptoms.

Other mechanisms for stroke include blood disorders, hypercoagulable states, latent neurosyphilis infection, inflammatory conditions of the blood vessels of the brain (vasculitis), and artery dissection.

It is extremely important to learn the warning signs of stroke. TIAs, as mentioned previously, are caused when blood flow is temporarily interrupted to an area of the brain. TIAs are commonly ignored because the symptoms are temporary and sometimes painless, or because the symptoms are attributed to old age or fatigue. One-third of all people who experience TIA may eventually have stroke. Additionally, your chance of having a stroke increases approximately ten-fold after you have had transient ischemic attack. It is very important to recognize TIA symptoms and to obtain medical treatment. TIAs may include sudden numbness or weakness of the face, arm or leg (especially when it occurs on one side of the body), sudden trouble seeing in one or both eyes, sudden confusion, and trouble speaking or understanding language. In addition, trouble walking, dizziness and loss of balance or coordination are common TIA symptoms. Also, sudden severe headache with no known cause may be a warning sign to stroke, and is most commonly seen in patients who have early cerebral hemorrhage.

Risk factors for stroke include hypertension, diabetes, peripheral vascular disease, coronary artery disease, age, smoking, lipid disorders and obesity. Some of these risk factors can be modified and some cannot.

Patient and community education is critical in ultimately providing efficient and effective stroke care. Chapter 7 will introduce further issues regarding diagnosis as well as primary and secondary treatment of stroke.

Chapter 3
EFFECTS OF STROKE

In the early hours of my stay at the hospital, the doctors knew I had had a stroke, and they knew roughly where it had occurred (the right side of my brain), but it took a couple of days for the full extent of the damage to reveal itself. My speech was slurred, I had a headache, and my left arm and leg seemed weak, but since the immediate objective was to stabilize me and let my body rest from the initial impact of the stroke, we didn't attempt too much physical or mental exertion. My son and daughter and their families arrived, and I received a couple of visits from friends and neighbors. I'm sure I wasn't much company, but it was good to know they were there.

One thing my family began to notice was that I had developed a tendency to only look to the right side of my hospital room, and that even when someone standing on my left spoke to me, I seldom turned my head toward them. When this was reported to my neurologist, he said that it was "left-side neglect," a common result of right-brain strokes.

Neglect is a perceptual disorder caused by damage to an

area near the back of the brain that processes sensory information. A person with neglect typically doesn't notice things on the stroke-involved side of the body. Not only do they not know there's something there, to them, there's no "there" there! Put one hand over your left eye and you get a general idea of what it's like. If you could also turn off the rest of your senses, you'd get an even closer approximation. Don't just imagine that you have trouble seeing or feeling things on the left—imagine that they don't exist! If your brain were telling you that the whole of the phenomenological world were contained within the area described by an imaginary line down the center of your head and the farthest thing you could see out of the peripheral vision of your right eye, it would be completely logical that you would not pay attention to things or people on your "left." To the friend or family member, neglect can seem odd or rude—like the patient is refusing to acknowledge them. But for the patient it makes complete sense. He's not ignoring you by choice, he's just not aware of you. It's not that the patient has lost her sight or her hearing—typically the organs of perception themselves are not affected by stroke. It's just that the information they are receiving is not being processed the way it used to.

My neglect was so severe that initially I was even unaware that I was partially paralyzed! Perhaps it was a blessing that I didn't know so I didn't have to worry about that during the early stages of recovery. When I did finally "notice" my weak left arm I asked, "can somebody move this thing, it's in my way." In extreme cases of neglect, the stroke patient may not even believe that his arm and leg belong to him. For a while I only half-jokingly called my arm, "Joe." Realizing what had happened to me, and understanding how the stroke had affected me, was a slow and gradual process.

The disabilities and dangers that accompany neglect are immediately apparent. In trying to walk or move about in a wheelchair, the patient might constantly run into the wall on the affected side. Or if outside, they may seem oblivious to oncoming traffic and begin to step into the street in front of a car. When tending to personal hygiene, why comb the left side of your hair or shave the left side of your face if, to you, there's nothing over there? This is an attention disorder of a remarkable kind, yet once you realize what has occurred there are numerous ways to compensate for this deficiency.

A term that has become a part of our family's vocabulary is **"cue,"** meaning to give verbal or physical instructions in order to elicit a desired behavior. Because of left-side neglect, I often need to be prompted to "look left." No two words have been more helpful—or more tiresome! "Eleanor, do you see my napkin?" "Look left." "I can't find the TV remote." "Look left." "Where's my toothbrush?" "Did you try looking left?" The annoyance of hearing that command over and over again has led me to try "cueing" myself. "Wish I had more to eat. Hmm, maybe I should check out the left side of my plate." Sometimes the way to a man's rehabilitation is through his stomach.

Speaking of food (which I dearly love), another result of the stroke was that for the first few days the left side of my throat was paralyzed, which made swallowing difficult at best. Every time I ate or drank something I coughed. Concerned that I not "aspirate" or breath food into my lungs, the doctor put me on a liquid, and then a soft diet, supplemented by an IV drip of sugar and vitamins. For a guy coming out of the fog of a stroke and longing to feel like his old self again, eating Jell-O and strained sweet potatoes didn't make me feel like I was on the fast track to recovery. Looming in the back of my mind was the fear that perhaps I would have to be fed through a tube, a depressing as well as unappetizing thought. A swallowing test was administered, which thankfully I passed, and I was allowed to ease my way back to a normal diet (well, normal for hospital food!).

Another symptom was that my speech was slurred. Having only recently moved to Florida from Virginia, I had not begun to lose my southern accent (nor do I suspect I ever will), but the medical staff and visitors found it unusually hard to understand me. Some stroke patients experience difficulty creating speech due to a condition called **aphasia**—most typically found in left-brain strokes. Subsequent work with a **speech therapist** revealed that my problem lay in the fact that, like other muscles on my left, the left side of my tongue was weak, and literally lagged behind as I formed words. I've worked at it for five years now, and still have difficulty pronouncing certain words.

According to *Family Guide to Stroke*[1] (a very helpful book published by the American Heart Association), common results of stroke include partial **paralysis,** neglect, slurred speech, unawareness and denial of the extent of one's condition, attention and short term memory problems, and a raft of possible personality and behavioral changes. Those are just the primary symptoms, and believe me I've experienced most of them. One also has to protect against complications setting in such as heart and blood vessel problems, urinary track infection and bladder control trouble, pneumonia and other respiratory disease, bed sores, stiffness, arthritis and depression. The whole focus of the first few days in the hospital after a stroke is the identification, treatment and prevention of these problems.

---

[1] *Family Guide to Stroke;* American Heart Association; Clarkson Potter, 1996.

Chapter 4
EARLY TREATMENT OF STROKE

Based on both my symptoms and the results of numerous tests, a complete diagnosis was finally determined. The neurologist explained to my family that either a blood clot or some other particle in my blood stream had clogged my right **carotid artery,** permanently blocking the blood flow to many of the brain cells normally fed by that vessel. Not every cell in the area was damaged, thanks in part to what's

All I heard was a stream of words pouring out of the mouth of a stranger in a white coat. "Mr. Prillaman," he said, "you have suffered an ischemic stroke caused by the occlusion of your right internal carotid artery, resulting in a large infarct that has affected significant areas of both the frontal and parietal lobes of your cerebral cortex." My only thought was, "Well, do you want to shoot me now, or am I already dead?"

called "collateral blood flow." Sensing a shortage of blood, other blood vessels take over and resume feeding the affected areas. When the full effect of the stroke had settled in, I was left with areas of my brain that no longer functioned, and the resultant disabilities.

I can't stress enough, however, that although I now have a general sense of what happened to me, when the doctor first described my condition all I heard was a stream of words pouring out of the mouth of a stranger in a white coat. The medical profession, like my own of education, is both plied and plagued with a special vocabulary of technical jargon that, while aiding the communication between experts, is in large part absolutely meaningless to the average person. "Mr. Prillaman," he said, "you have suffered an **ischemic stroke** caused by the **occlusion** of your right internal **carotid artery,** resulting in a large **infarct** that has affected significant areas of both the **frontal** and **parietal lobes** of your **cerebral cortex.**" My only thought was, "Well, do you want to shoot me now, or am I already dead?"

Frankly, I don't remember ever being told the simple facts about what had happened to me. There were bits and pieces of scientific jargon, and I suspect my family understood the situation before I did, but my unshakable impression is that in the medical world there is an extreme lack of comprehensible information given to the very people who are most desperate to know what's going on. Sure, I was told by a number of physicians that I had had a stroke, and that it was a major one—the kind that is sometimes fatal. I understood that it was a right-brain attack, affecting the left side of my body which is now partially paralyzed. But clearly I would have benefited from a more straightforward explanation about my condition, the cause, and the prognosis. As it was, I was still searching for an exact understanding of my situation well into the rehabilitation process months later.

As I gradually became more aware of my disabilities, I went through the process that is often used when encountering a child that needs special education services. One morning I awoke earlier than usual (a miracle in itself since I love to sleep in and normally can't even hold a conversation

Frankly, I don't remember ever being told the simple facts about what had happened to me. In the medical world there is an extreme lack of comprehensible information given to the very people who are most desperate to know what's going on. Clearly, I would have benefited from a more straightforward explanation about my condition, the cause, and the prognosis.

before I have a cup of coffee, a cigarette, and the morning paper). I began to wrestle with the question of how you would classify my condition. Was I disabled or handicapped or both, and was it mild, moderate or severe? As a special education administrator one tries to diagnose the student's major handicap in order to prescribe the proper educational placement. I went through the list of possibilities: mentally retarded, physically handicapped, emotionally disturbed, brain damaged, multiply handicapped.... As I thought this through I became filled with the old anger I used to feel when others would attempt to label kids. Yes, I am brain-damaged—that's what a stroke does to one—and seriously so. And yes, I am now a bit retarded—but fortunately it is a mild condition. And certainly I am physically handicapped. But most importantly I am still Doug Prillaman, and will not suffer anyone to reduce me or others to a mere label.

One of the first treatments they gave me was to put me on a blood thinner. Since they had determined that my stroke was caused by some sort of clot, they wanted to make sure my blood was now flowing freely. Of course, being on a blood thinner means you have to be careful not to cut yourself, so shaving was out for the first few days and I began to take on a certain Grizzly Adams appearance. They also were monitoring the oxygen levels in my blood to make sure my brain was getting all the nutrients it needed. For several days I wore an oxygen tube in my nose which was quite an aggravation when it came time to eat. During this time, there was also the constant drip of glucose to supplement my diet.

From time to time I had to take **respiratory therapy** to keep my lungs clear. Since I spent most of the time lying down, they had to make sure I wasn't getting a buildup of fluid.

As I came out of the shock of the initial attack, I started being aware of pain—and sometimes a lot of it. When my head wasn't hurting, my body was. Further tests revealed that the headaches were due in part to the damaged part of my brain being swollen and it took several days of medication for that to subside. The body pain, especially across my shoulders, would last for several months.

Since they had me hooked up to all manner of monitors and tubes, they wanted me to be fairly immobile, which meant being subjected to the indignity of a bed pan and a urinal. Having grown up in the country, I was familiar with keeping a pot in the room. (In my house, a "pecan" was a nut, but a "pee-can" was what you kept under the bed.) But having to use such a device while lying down was a whole other trick. After a few accidents, the nurse fitted me with a thing called a "Texas Catheter" (and I use the term "fitted" loosely). Whatever cowboy invented the Texas **Cath** should be strung up on the nearest tree. We tried all different sizes and brands, but when all was said (mostly cursing) and done (mostly leaking), I went back to the urinal.

Maybe it was the medication, or the countless times they wheeled me down some hall to a different part of the hospital for more tests, or maybe it was the stroke itself, but I often felt confused about where I was. To add to that, one day they moved me to an entirely different floor. My wife later explained that since I had stabilized, they were able to move me from the **critical care** unit to what they called **progressive care.** Of course, a new floor meant a different room, different nurses and different aides, but it was a relief to be told that I was making progress and was out of danger of an immediate recurrence.

Once in progressive care, I began having visitors from another group of specialists. A **Dietician** met with me to make sure that, now that I was off the glucose drip, I was getting enough nourishment. A **physical therapist** came in a couple of times to assess the extent of my loss of use of my left leg and arm. She took me through a number of initial tests, but then seemed to disappear. Neither my family nor I knew enough to recognize that this was not necessarily a good sign.

I was allowed to sit up more often, and with help and a wheelchair, I was able to explore my hall and get to the bathroom to shave. Little did I know at that time that a wheelchair would become such a permanent part of my life.

After several days, we began to hear talk that I might be moved yet again. The hospital was no longer the place for me and the **neurologist** and physical therapist were consulting about my options after being discharged. Depending on the severity of the stroke and the resultant disabilities, a patient is usually sent to either a **rehabilitation facility,** a **nursing home,** or, in the best-case scenario, back to his own home. I didn't know how bad off I was, but clearly they determined that there was the possibility of recovery of some or all of my lost function, so a nursing home was ruled out. Going home would have given me the most peace of mind, but the sense was that a rigorous program of various therapies was called for, and that these could best be provided in a residential rehabilitation hospital. With that decision made, my wife inquired as to when and how the transfer would be affected. For 48 hours she asked questions— "Which rehab facility was best?" "What paperwork would be needed to gain admission?" "Would insurance cover the costs?" "How and when would the actual move, itself, occur?" And for 48 hours she was told only, "We'll get back to you." Then one afternoon out of the clear blue an ambulance driver just shows up at my bedside and says, "Let's go!" As luck would have it, it was one of the few times Eleanor wasn't there at the hospital with me. Thankfully, our daughter-in-law, who happened to be visiting at the moment, was able to throw all my worldly belongings into a couple of grocery bags and we were out the door! Ten minutes later I was on a gurney being rolled out of the ambulance and into my new home-away-from-home, a residential rehabilitation facility.

Chapter 5
ADMISSION TO THE REHAB HOSPITAL

T he folks at the rehab hospital seemed as surprised to see me as I was to see them. Apparently they had received some vague notice that I was coming, but no one had any idea when. As luck would have it, I arrived unannounced just before the afternoon nursing staff change. As my family and I waited in the hallway (I on a gurney they had used to transport me from the hospital), I think we all began to wonder: what in the world have we gotten ourselves into now?

At this rehab facility, the staff works three eight-hour shifts, and the turnover between teams is the epitome of organized chaos. As one team is trying to finish up their work and close out their paperwork, another is coming in and trying to get a jump on things before the usual mania ensues. Pill pushers (what I called the nurses who handle the medication) are busy organizing their "pharmacy on wheels," **charge nurses** (a stern-looking breed who seem to serve as both traffic cops and camp managers) are digging in or out of a pile of paperwork, **L.P.N.s** and **R.N.s** in color-coded smocks (a code I could never seem to crack) hurried behind closed doors to dictate the day's proceedings into tape recorders, while **nurses' aides** scurried around tidying up the common areas and generally looking too busy to be interrupted.

Pill pushers (what I called the nurses who handle the medication) are busy organizing their "pharmacy on wheels," charge nurses (a stern-looking breed who seem to serve as both traffic cops and camp managers) are digging in or out of a pile of paperwork, L.P.N.s and R.N.s in color-coded smocks (a code I could never seem to crack) hurried behind closed doors to dictate the day's proceedings, while nurses' aides scurried around looking too busy to be interrupted.

Someone finally figured out who I was and where I belonged and rolled me into a semi-private room. The accommodations were nice enough. Luckily the facility had recently undergone a renovation. In a relatively small space they had fit two over-sized hospital beds, complete with the requisite tubes and monitors and electrical curiosities, plus two armoires, two bedside chairs, and a shared bathroom and sink. I had a window that looked out on a small retention pond, the sometimes noisy home of various frogs, bugs and wading birds.

My roommate—the first of many—was either asleep or

heavily sedated, and didn't have much to say. I imagine he was wondering what I was doing invading his space, at the same time that I was wondering what kind of person he was and what he was in there for.

This rehab hospital, part of a large chain with locations throughout the country, apparently prided itself on being a "restraint-free" facility. As they were helping me to bed, they proudly mentioned that they didn't believe in strapping patients into their beds or buckling them into wheel chairs. What they neglected to tell me was that everything in that whole darned building was alarmed. If you got up out of your bed, an alarm went off. If you got up out of your wheelchair, an alarm went off. If you opened the wrong door or window, another alarm went off. What benefit to one's dignity there may have been in not being restrained was certainly tempered by the din of beeps and buzzes that accompanied your every move. Multiply that array of noises times the number of patients in the hospital and you can imagine that no one—neither the staff nor the patients—gets much rest.

After the hubbub of my arrival died down, the extent of the facility's unpreparedness to receive me began to reveal itself. Every service they offer—from medical care to the various rehabilitative therapies to simply getting something to eat—is approved and coordinated by an on-site **case manager.** But since they didn't know when I was coming, there was no case manager there to officially admit me, and it was the start of the weekend, to boot. So for the first three days of my tenure it was basically up to my wife and family to figure out how things worked around there and who was who and what was where.

To add insult to injury, my chart that came with me from the hospital did not use my preferred name, Doug, but my first name—Floyd—which no one had called me in 50 years. So to the stream of nurses and aides who came to my beside and inquired, "how do you feel, Floyd?" I could only answer, "not myself."

Once the case manager arrived and I was properly admitted, things began to settle into a daily routine....

Chapter 6
LIFE AS A LONG-TERM INPATIENT

The start of my rehabilitation program was further delayed by a common occurrence in any group living situation—the common cold. Actually, the not-so-common flu, accompanied by an ill-timed urinary tract infection. Although it delayed the start of my therapy sessions, it did give me a chance to get to know the ins and outs of the facility.

The rehab hospital was part of a large chain run by a for-profit corporation, and this combination of healthcare and a bottom line orientation resulted in a predictably institutional atmosphere. Although decorated nicely and populated by a largely pleasant staff, the whole operation was run like a factory. Everything ran on a schedule, and that schedule was apparently handed down by an invisible but all-seeing technocrat. What time you ate, what time you slept, when you could take a shower, when you had therapy, when you could have visitors was all according to schedule. For a guy who had chosen early retirement to rid his life of any schedule, this required numerous unwelcome adjustments.

41

A typical day meant up at 7:00 (something I hadn't done since the Army), breakfast at 8:00 (without the consciousness-restoring benefit of a newspaper and a cigarette), and by 8:30 I found myself—still groggy and often grumpy—at my first therapy session. Further, I was denied several of the inalienable rights of retirement: the morning walk, the afternoon nap, and cocktail hour.

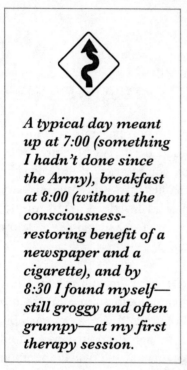

A typical day meant up at 7:00 (something I hadn't done since the Army), breakfast at 8:00 (without the consciousness-restoring benefit of a newspaper and a cigarette), and by 8:30 I found myself—still groggy and often grumpy—at my first therapy session.

The physical environment was nice enough. Most patients shared a double room located down one of several long hallways. At the intersection of the hallways were various common areas such as a public restroom, a lounge or a dining hall. Across the other side of the main lobby were the rooms set aside for various therapies. One labeled **"PT"** was full of low, padded platforms, walls of mirrors and odd-looking workout equipment. Another designated **"OT"** contained rows of tables which held what appeared to be various child's toys and puzzles. The most curious of the rooms was behind a closed door marked "Work Hardening." I never found out what that meant, but all I knew was I had retired to avoid work and didn't want anything to do with something called "hardening."

Because of the regimented life of the hospital, it was weeks before I had the time to wander all the halls and see everything in the facility, but it was all pretty much the same—long corridors of rooms filled with broken or disabled people, connected by nurses' stations, staff offices and uninviting patient lounges. I did make careful note of where all the exits were in case I had to effect an escape.

One guiding principle of my pre-stroke daily life was that the fewer people I had to see before the second cup of coffee the better. However here I found myself wheeled into a common dining room filled with strangers, most of whom were in similar or worse shape than I. Since most were too ill or too unhappy to offer much small talk, you were left with the strange sensation of sitting alone, crowded elbow-to-elbow with mute strangers. Your food arrived on a cafeteria tray delivered by workers who were alternately oddly sullen or annoyingly upbeat.

Despite these drawbacks, the motivation to show up for breakfast was high since if you missed this feeding it would be four more hours before a tasty morsel would pass your lips. And the food was surprisingly delicious. How the cooks were able to turn out such good food from an institutional kitchen I'll never know, but there was a continuous supply of appetizing and nourishing food.

After breakfast, it was down the hall to your first therapy session of the day. Most of us had three back-to-back one-hour sessions without a break—a schedule designed in part to move a lot of people through the system and in part to build up your stamina after being off your feet and in a hospital bed for several days or even weeks. Then it was lunch, and the therapies started all over again. I was typically finished by 4:00 or 4:30, and wheeled my way back to my room in hopes of a restorative snooze before dinner. However, since most of the staff was at that point making preparations for dinner, it was nigh on impossible to find anybody who would take a moment to help you out of your wheelchair and up onto your bed. Instead, you were lined up outside the dining hall to await the dinner bell. Thus, the period of the day that would normally involve a refreshing nap or a bracing round of cocktails with friends held forth nothing more than a respite from physical exertion and a sometimes lengthy period of isolation as you joined the scores of other patients slumped in their wheelchairs from exhaustion—a sight which added mightily to the general sense of malaise in the place.

After dinner there was a brief period of free time, but most of us just went back to our rooms and waited for the nurse's aide to come help us get into bed. The evening hours might be interrupted by a visit from the pill pusher, or, on alternating nights, an offer to help you take a shower or sponge bath, but mainly you lay in your bed watching TV (or listening to the blare of your roommate's TV) and trying to figure out how you got here and how you were going to get out. Sleeping became the only thing that seemed like your old life, yet before you knew it, it was morning and the routine started all over again.

Chapter 7
CURRENT PRACTICES IN TREATMENT OF STROKE
Dr. S. James Shafer, M.D.

I t wasn't many years ago that the management and treatment of stroke was very limited. Before current research into the understanding of stroke mechanisms and the advent of "clot-busting" drugs, patients with stroke were simply hospitalized and monitored for progressive symptoms with hopes that they would stabilize. In short, stroke patients were not considered highly rehabilitative.

In the past decade, there have been revolutionary changes in the treatment and management of

One of the most important factors in stroke management is early detection. A person experiencing stroke symptoms should contact 911 or go to the emergency room immediately. Time is of the essence.

stroke. A primary focus has been on prevention and risk reduction. Plus, with the evolutionary concept of "brain attack," there has been an increased awareness of the necessity for acute care immediately after the onset of stroke symptoms. Improved functional outcomes are known to occur in patients who receive early, aggressive and comprehensive neurorehabilitation.

One of the most important factors in stroke management is early detection. A person experiencing stroke symptoms should contact 911 or go to the emergency room immediately. Time is of the essence, as there is a certain window within which a patient must be evaluated in order to receive medications that potentially can reverse the deficits of stroke.

Once a patient has recognized stroke symptoms and reported to an acute care center, a comprehensive neurological examination is undertaken. Higher cortical function testing will allow the doctor to assess areas of the brain that control language and cognitive processing. The examination will also evaluate primary functions of vision, swallowing and speech production. Additionally, there will be an elemental examination of motor strength and sensation. In virtually all circumstances, the physician will be able to localize the area of the brain which has been affected by stroke.

To further aid in the evaluation of stroke, patients may undergo diagnostic testing. The first test typically performed is a **CT scan** (or **cat scan**), an x-ray of the brain which is predominantly used to determine whether or not there has been bleeding into the brain. If there is a hemorrhage, treatment options are limited, and mostly center around managing blood pressure, vital signs and monitoring for symptoms of decreased level of consciousness.

It is not uncommon for a CT scan to be normal in the presence of an early ischemic stroke. CT scan's resolution is not optimal for detecting stroke, and in the early minutes to hours of stroke, tissue swelling and changes in nerve cells have not progressed enough for CT scan to detect. New imaging techniques are being utilized to more readily assess the extent of stroke damage and to determine what part of the brain may be most susceptible to further damage.

If the patient has been able to reach the emergency room within two hours and has had a complete stroke evaluation within three hours, many hospitals will consider the patient a candidate for TPA. TPA (Tissue Plasminogen Activator) is a recently approved "clot-busting" medication. Each hospital has criteria which include or exclude patients for receiving TPA, and these criteria are discussed

If the patient has been able to reach the emergency room within two hours and has had a complete stroke evaluation within three hours, many hospitals will consider the patient a candidate for TPA, a recently approved "clot-busting" medication.

with the family and the patient at the time of presentation. If it is determined that the patient might benefit from TPA, they will receive a portion of the medication in the emergency room, and the balance after they are transferred to intensive care. Thereafter, monitoring and management of vital signs and neurological function will continue during the next one to two days.

Once the patient has been stabilized and acute management has been undertaken, focus should then be turned to the family and caregivers. This is a very stressful and traumatic time for them as well, and they should be informed regarding all aspects of acute care. The risks and benefits of various medications and treatments should be explained, followed by a realistic discussion of possible outcomes.

The first 24-48 hours after a stroke are very unpredictable. Although the patient may appear stable, there still can be dramatic changes in neurological function. The family should have a good understanding of the patient's deficits, especially if there are language difficulties and neglect, as they must be given strategies for communicating with the patient.

Other treatments of stroke include the use of intravenous anticoagulant medications (such as Heparin™), especially in the case of patients who have a high risk of cardiac embolism. Patients who had a stroke as a consequence of a recent myocardial infarction (heart attack) may also be placed on IV Heparin™. Antiplatelet agents such as clopidogrel (Plavix™) and dipyridamole/aspirin (Aggrenox™) affect the "stickiness" of the platelets which form blood clots and are used in some acute stroke management scenarios.

The recent introduction of the term "brain attack" to describe stroke emphasizes the urgency with which one must respond to stroke symptoms. Past studies have demonstrated that 50-70% of patients don't get to the hospital until 24 or more hours after the onset of symptoms. One must understand that a stroke or brain attack is as much of a medical emergency as a heart attack. Once the patient has been managed through the acute stages of stroke, they are commonly referred to rehabilitation.

Rehabilitation is a comprehensive team effort that involves **physical therapy, occupational thera-py, speech therapy** and **cognitive thera-py,** all led by a physician specially trained in stroke rehabilitation. At this point in stroke treatment, an outside support system becomes very important. Patients who have strong family support

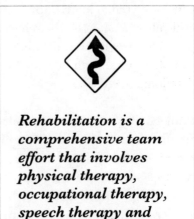

Rehabilitation is a comprehensive team effort that involves physical therapy, occupational therapy, speech therapy and cognitive therapy, all led by a physician specially trained in stroke rehabilitation.

in place fare much better in what is often a long and complex rehabilitative process. **Caregivers** and family need to be actively involved in all phases of the patient's rehab and should inquire about being present during critical times of therapy. When the patient is transferred home, the caregivers and family will become actively involved in helping with the patient's continuing rehabilitation and daily needs.

Monitoring for **depression** is of importance with patients who have suffered stroke. Post-stroke depression is quite common, and not identifying and addressing it can hinder the patient's continued progress and delay his recovery. Pre-stroke personality plays a significant role in illness behavior, and each patient will react differently. Some will require more and some less motivation to proceed with the rehabilitative process. Behavior should be critically evaluated by the rehabilitative team as well as the patient's caregivers and family so that there might be a complete understanding of the patient's physical and emotional needs.

Primary and secondary stroke prevention techniques are key in both preventing the initial stroke event and reducing the risk of recurrence. Primary prevention revolves around reducing risk factors, some of which can be modified and some of which cannot. The patient's age, gender and genetic makeup, of course, cannot be modified. But factors such as blood pressure, high cholesterol, obesity, sedentary lifestyle, excessive use of alcohol and tobacco can all be modified in order to reduce the chances of stroke.

Medications which affect the way the blood forms clots are sometimes used in the prevention of stroke. Coumadin™, an anticoagulant which has a limited role in stroke prevention, is utilized in patients with cardiac arrhythmia such as atrial fibrillation, and in those with septal defects or a history of ventricular (heart) aneurysm. Coumadin™ may also be used in some cases of severe narrowing (stenosis) of intra-cerebral vessels of the brain. The qualification for any one particular drug is varied among patients and depends upon multiple factors determined by the treating physician.

Unfortunately, there is no medication which will guarantee that a stroke will never occur. It cannot be stressed enough that risk factor reduction is extremely important in the prevention of stroke, and that patients should seek regular visits with their primary care physician. For example, nearly half of all strokes that occur in the United States could be eliminated with appropriate blood pressure control.

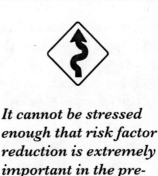

It cannot be stressed enough that risk factor reduction is extremely important in the prevention of stroke, and that patients should seek regular visits with their primary care physician. Nearly half of all strokes could be eliminated with appropriate blood pressure control.

The treatment and management of stroke are continuously evolving through the efforts of research. For many years, the only effective stroke treatment was rehabilitation, and barring that, nursing home placement. However, early detection of stroke symptoms and new medications for the treatment of acute stroke are revolutionizing the outcome of this devastating event. There is a strong interest in neuronal (nerve cell) protection, and neuroprotective agents are being studied to prevent further cell death. New research is also underway to learn how to protect those neurons which are "stunned" by stroke, in hopes that with re-perfusion (the return of blood flow) there will be less cell death, and thus fewer physical deficits. With continued research and ongoing patient education as to the warning signs, symptoms and mechanisms of stroke, thousands of people are working to reduce the number of strokes which occur in the United States annually.

Chapter 8
EARLY ATTEMPTS AT REHABILITATION

My initial experience of rehabilitation therapy was that I was rolled into a large room abuzz with activity as a meager handful of therapists struggled to give their attention to what seemed like an army of invalids. An hour in that room consisted of about 20 minutes of work and 40 minutes of waiting around. Before I knew it, I was being rolled off to some other end of the building to be alternately attended to and ignored by another equally-harried staff.

The goal of rehabilitation is to help the patient regain lost functions, maintain those they still have, and retrain them to do old activities in new ways.

Behind the scenes, it turns out there was some method to the apparent madness. It was later explained to me that the rehabilitation process was run by a team of people, all working under the direction of my neurologist. Their goal, as I came to understand it, was to help me regain lost functions, maintain those I still had, and to retrain me to do old activities in new ways. Although in some cases rehabilitation can result in a complete restoration of previous abilities, for most people it's about adapting to your deficits and recovering as much independence as possible.

The classic rehabilitation team might be made up of as many as a dozen different people, starting with the patient, the primary care **physician,** and the patient's family or main caregivers. To that core might be added numerous therapists and specialists whose job it is to concentrate on one specific area of your rehabilitation, under the leadership and coordination of the lead doctor.

Physical therapists are mainly concerned with getting you back on your feet, walking as best you can, and lower body issues. **Occupational therapists,** despite the term, don't have anything to do with your current or former occupation, but with restoring your ability to do the typical "activities of daily living," or **"ADLs."** As such, their work seems to focus on the use of the upper part of your body, such as dressing, bathing, eating and generally getting through the day. **Speech therapists** help you not just with speaking, but with any communication deficit and the cognitive functions that support them. **Recreational therapy** is not all fun and games, but it is an additional opportunity to sharpen your mental and motor skills by activities normally thought of as hobbies or play. **Psychologists** can help deal with emotional issues that arise, such as the depression that may result from coming to grips with your disabilities and the changes they are bringing to your life and those you love. **Vocational therapists** can help you prepare to return to work, and **social workers** might assist with other issues involved in returning to society after your stroke. Add to that a **dietitian** or **nutritionist** plus a raft of nurses and aides, and you've got a rehabilitation team.

Not every patient needs help from all of these people. Based on your primary physician's prognosis and evaluation, a rehabilitation strategy is drawn up and the necessary specialists are brought in to do their part. From that point on, they meet regularly as a team to discuss your progress and make any adjustments to the program they deem necessary.

On paper, a rehabilitation team is a good thing, but in practice things may not run so smoothly. During my stay in rehab I had five different physical therapists, three occupational therapists and a host of assistants and volunteers, each of whom seemed to have a different way of helping me do the same tasks. Retraining your brain to walk is a difficult enough process without getting conflicting instructions from different therapists. But in the world of corporate health care, you apparently have to put up with all manner of less-than-desirable service. Heaven help the person in rehab who doesn't have a competent doctor and a conscientious caregiver.

STROKE

Chapter 9
THE ROLE OF THE PHYSICAL THERAPIST

Although at the time I didn't recognize it as such, my experience with physical therapy had begun in the hospital just days after my stroke. My son reminded me that a therapist had visited the room several times, bringing with her a large rolling mirror. Considering all that I was going through, my appearance was not among my immediate concerns. However the mirror served a different purpose other than reflecting on my lack of sartorial splendor.

Since the stroke occurred in the right half of my brain, the physical deficits I experienced were largely on the left. In addition to the left-neglect discussed earlier, I also tended to slump to the left, "weak" side when sitting up. My muscles had not been damaged, it's just that the signals from my brain to the left side of my body were not getting through. When the therapist came to my room, she asked me to sit on the edge of the bed and look at myself in the mirror. It took a while before I noticed it, but I was clearly slouching to the left. Repeated attempts at sitting up straight slowly began to pay off, yet initially it took the mirror to help me realize that I was slumped over.

Although a healthy person hardly thinks about it, centering one's weight is critical to sitting, standing and walking, and is used in nearly every action not performed from a prone position. It was several days before I began to hold myself up straight without being reminded, but regaining this ability was one of the first proofs of the value of PT.

Physical therapy begins with an evaluation of the patient's disabilities, followed by an assessment of how much function can likely be regained. Next, a strategy is laid out and goals are set. Periodic reviews of the patient's progress determine successive elements of the program.

The formal process of physical therapy begins with an evaluation of the type and extent of the patient's physical disabilities, leading to an initial assessment of how much function can likely be regained. Next, a strategy is laid out and goals are set. From there, periodic reviews of the patient's progress determine successive elements of his or her program.

Although I was understandably anxious to work on learning how to walk again, my therapist first devoted a considerable amount of our time together to massaging and flexing my left hand, arm, shoulder and leg. She would bend and straighten my arm, massage and extend my fingers (which had begun to atrophy and curl inward into a fist), and rotate my leg at the hip, knee and ankle. These "range-of-motion" exercises are designed to keep any paralyzed limbs from stiffening or contracting, a condition that can make more active exercise all the more difficult and potentially painful. This passive activity also serves to stimulate the brain in still-healthy areas not normally used for this purpose. With repetition, the brain can learn to compensate for deficiencies in stroke-damaged areas and "rewire" itself in order to accomplish tasks using alternate parts of the brain.

Next up was getting up! Moving from the bed to your wheel chair or from either to a standing position is called "transferring." For many stroke victims, transferring is the gateway to mobility. In my first efforts, it took all of my concentration, two therapists and a contraption around my waist called a "gait belt." The belt gives the therapist something to grab onto in case you start to fall. As a wardrobe item it's definitely not my style, but many times I was glad they grabbed the belt instead of my arm or shoulder, or worse, let me fall to the ground.

My job was to look down to make sure that both of my feet were planted squarely on the floor, slip to the edge of my seat, give an audible count so that the therapist knew when I was going to make my move, and then, with a rocking motion, lean forward until my nose was over my toes and, pushing up with my right hand and right leg, struggle to a standing position. I'll confess I fell back into a sitting position more than once until finally, with no little tugging by the therapist on the gait belt, I was able to straighten up and remain standing.

The sense of victory that accompanied this achievement was quickly replaced with a sense of panic—would my legs hold me, or would I topple over? Thankfully the therapists had been through this many times before and were ready to steady me should I go wobbly. After verbally reviewing the steps involved in successfully standing, they helped me sit back down and regain my composure. We must have performed that maneuver three or four times before I grew tired and asked for a break.

After learning that I could trust my legs for short periods of time, we worked on building up my balance and endurance. Exercises such as shifting my weight from side to side, shallow knee bends, and leaning over while sitting were prescribed to build up my stamina. One day the therapist brought in a large beach ball and had me try to catch it or bat it away while standing. Although these were just sneaky ways to get me to make the kind of spontaneous corrections to my balance typically required by walking down the street, at least it was a change of pace and a little taste of the old days when I used to coach basketball at the junior high.

Other exercises were performed on a raised gymnastic mat. While my therapist had to run off to work with another patient, I was to do 20 or 30 repetitions of things called "trunk rolls" and "bridges," exercises designed to strengthen my back, hips and buttocks. I found the mat much more suited to napping than exercising, but I generally did my duty after a brief period of procrastination.

Although walking comes as second nature for most healthy individuals, those who have suffered brain-related injuries often have to learn to walk all over again. Imagine looking down at your arm or leg and saying, "move," and nothing happens. You're thinking "move forward," but you might as well be talking to a rock. In my case, it was because the area of my brain that normally controlled the motor functions of the left side of my body had gone without blood and oxygen for so long that the cells finally quit sending and receiving messages to those muscle groups. The lines of communication from the brain to the leg had been cut, and no amount of wishing otherwise was going to change things. But walking again was my main goal in rehabilitation, and I was determined to do so.

When the physical therapist thought I was ready to attempt the first few steps, she devised a system that involved giving me a series of voice commands or "cues." Typically she would say something like, "cane" (move the cane forward with my right hand), "lean" (shift my weight so that most of it is on the cane and my stronger right leg), "left" (move my left foot forward), followed by "right." At the beginning, many was the time that the therapist said "left" and absolutely nothing happened. After much repetition, I was able to get some movement in my left leg, but often not enough to really call it a "step." The first trick we tried was putting a sock over my left shoe so that it more easily slid across the floor. (Later I was prescribed a device called an **"AFO,"** short for "ankle-foot orthosis," which helped keep "ole lefty" from dragging behind.)

With all my concentration being focused on my left leg, the therapist noticed that I was taking very small steps with my strong, right leg. In order to remind me to increase the length of my stride, she changed the command "right" to "through," which significantly increased the amount of ground I could cover with each step.

At first we did most of my walking on the parallel bars. Walking between them gave me a certain sense of confidence that if I fell I could catch myself on the bars. After walking back and forth between the bars, moving out onto the open floor didn't seem quite so frightening.

Once on the floor, it was critical that the therapist walk right beside me and hold on to my gait belt. In fact, because I'm a big guy, it took two therapists. We also experimented with a variety of canes. The typical straight cane is the easiest to handle, but when you're starting out it doesn't provide much support. I tried two-, three- and four-legged canes. The larger the base, the more the stability, but the easier to get tangled up in. We ended up working mostly with a low profile quad cane, providing the added support of four legs but with a smaller "footprint." As I got more proficient, I was able to walk with only one therapist holding on. Later, I could walk with the therapist only providing audible cues and following alongside.

After getting up some confidence walking on a flat, smooth surface, they had me walk on varying kinds of carpet and even on grass and uneven ground outside. We went up and down stairs and ramps, did laps around the rehab facility, and in the latter stages focused on working up some speed and developing a more natural gait.

Walking smoothly and quickly is both exhilarating and a bit frightening. To this day, I still have to keep practicing, and I always make sure that my wife or someone else is walking alongside in case I lose my balance.

During the early phase of my physical therapy, there were some on my rehabilitative team who didn't think I was ever going to be able to walk again. My left-side neglect was so bad, and my semi-paralysis so severe, that some were of a mind to release me from the rehab hospital without having taken a single step. To my good fortune, one therapist said she thought she had seen some signs that I might still have a chance, and recommended to the team leader that they keep trying. How happy I was—and how surprised they were—when the very next day I took my first step. Thanks to the talent and perseverance of my physical therapists, I was able to learn new ways to compensate, new ways to walk with a cane and an aide, and eventually, new ways to live.

STROKE

Chapter 10
THE ROLE OF THE OCCUPATIONAL THERAPIST

Occupational therapy goes hand in had with physical therapy, but for some reason I could never get as excited about "OT" as "PT." One reason is that most of the exercises they had us do seemed so disconnected from everyday life—an odd thing, considering OT is supposed to be about restoring your ability to do the "activities of daily living."

A typical OT session involved putting plastic rings over a wooden pole, running a hoop over a wire course, working puzzles and all manner of childish games. When I questioned why we were doing these sorts of exercises, I was told that these devices had been specifically designed by occupational therapists to help develop upper body motor skills. Maybe so, but I constantly wondered if the same benefits couldn't be achieved by working with more adult objects such as turning the pages of a newspaper, pushing buttons on the TV remote control, and pouring the cold beverage of your choice over ice. Now there are some activities I'd like to be "occupied" with!

The prognosis for a person undergoing occupational

therapy is in part related to how much use of their upper body they retained after the stroke. Luckily, in my case, the stroke affected my left side, not my dominant right side. The unimpaired use of my right had allowed me to feed myself, grasp objects, use a pen, etc. But any task that required two hands was literally beyond my reach.

About the time I began OT, I began experiencing tremendous pain in my stroke-related left shoulder. I couldn't move it, and I didn't have much sensation, but I sure could still feel pain. One theory was that since the muscles in my left arm were no longer being told by my brain how to do their job, the unsupported weight of my limp arm was literally pulling my arm right out of the shoulder socket, similar to a dislocation. Another theory was that I had a condition known as "frozen shoulder," where the shoulder joint gets so inflamed that you experience severe stiffness and pain. More range-of-motion exercises were prescribed for the stiffness, but any sort of movement at all only increased the pain! Welcome to the Catch-22 world of rehabilitation therapy.

Although the therapists tried various liniments, heating pads and even immersed my arm in a hot container of dried corn kernels, it would be months before I was able to find relief from the pain. You can imagine that I was not an eager participant when it came to what I saw as occupational therapy's childish games. Several times I suggested that we quit OT and let me have an additional hour in PT working on my walking, but my requests seemed to fall on deaf ears. Ironically, my OT therapist was one of my favorite people I worked with, but I just couldn't seem to get them to change their system. Later, after I was released from the rehab hospital and began receiving in-home treatments, I was blessed with an occupational therapist who taught me all manner of helpful methods for getting out of bed, dressing and doing chores around the house. To this day, I still use many of the techniques and tips she shared with me.

STROKE

Chapter 11
THE ROLE OF THE SPEECH THERAPIST

S peech therapy" is a bit of a misnomer, as the field is concerned with much more than just how one talks. The more formal term, "speech-language pathology," suggests the broader scope of the science with includes all of the motor, sensory and cognitive skills involved in communicating.

Communication is a complex process that involves several different parts of the brain. In most people, speech and language are typically controlled in the left, more dominant **hemisphere** of the brain. If a stroke involves the part

Speech therapy is concerned with much more than just how one talks. It addresses all of the motor, sensory and cognitive skills involved in communicating.

of the brain nearest the top of the spinal cord, known as the **brain stem,** messages from the brain to the mouth might come out garbled due to a problem similar to crossed wires. If the stroke occurs above that in an area known as the **temporal lobe,** some people develop a condition called **Wernicke's Aphasia,** which basically means that, although they may hear fine, they have trouble understanding what is being said to them. The problem sometimes even causes them to speak in a scrambled manner, using the wrong word in an otherwise normally-constructed sentence, or even talking a kind of nonsense that has the rhythm of normal speech but where the words are jumbled. Finally, if the stroke occurs in the front portion of the brain known as the **frontal lobe,** it may affect your "motor cortex," the area which controls not only your large motor skills such as walking, but even the movement of your mouth, lips and tongue.

Thankfully, speech therapy can help people with many of these deficiencies, known as **"aphasia."** And because the process of communicating involves so many diverse parts of the brain, a stroke victim may be able to communicate in any number of alternative ways. Some who, after a stroke, cannot talk, have no trouble at all with writing or using gestures to convey their thoughts. Some with speech problems find that they can sing their words and get them out fine. Problems of comprehension, or "sensory aphasia," are much more difficult to resolve, but sometimes both therapy and the passage of time can improve the situation.

In my case, the stroke affected the right part of my fontal lobe that contains the motor cortex for the left side of my body. Not only were my left arm and left leg affected, but all of the left side of me, including the left side of my mouth, lips and tongue. My problems were not with forming thoughts clearly, but with forming the actual syllables that make up words. The same muscular problem is what caused me to temporarily have trouble swallowing, or **"dysphagia."** With training from my very talented speech therapist and a lot of concentration, I'm now able to deal with both.

My therapist also helped me with various cognitive problems. Due to my left-side neglect, I would typically start reading from the middle of the page in a book—it just didn't occur to me to look further than what seemed to me to be the edge of the page. She would also have me scan a page of print and draw a circle around, for example, all the "Ms." Invariably, I would only see those Ms on the right hand half of the page. She would also have me read passages aloud and then tell her what they meant. Often, it seemed like nonsense to me since I typically read only the right hand half of the page. By drawing a bright yellow line down the left hand margin of the page, she was able to "cue me" to keep scanning to the left until I saw the yellow line. After much practice, it became second nature to make sure I looked all the way to the left before I started reading.

The speech pathologist and I worked on what seemed like simple things, for example, telling time. With a digital clock which displayed the time in numerals, I was usually fine; but with a typical wall clock or watch, I usually got it wrong. You guessed it—I wasn't noticing the clock hands if they were pointing to a number on the left half of the clock. Although I hadn't worn a watch for years, she made me get one so I could practice.

I fared a little bit better on math problems—she used

coins as well as written numerals to check that part of my cognition. But, as is typical with a lot of stroke patients, I had problems with sequencing things in the right order. Initially, it was hard for me to remember which holidays came first in a calendar year, and I had difficulty keeping historical events in the proper order. It became a daily routine for me to have to tell her the day and date of the week, and we often worked with a calendar to get things in the proper order.

My speech therapist was one of my favorites, and I looked forward to working with her every day. However, on the way in and out of her office I would usually pass other patients, many of whom had more severe cognition problems than I. It should have made me grateful, but being surrounded by others with so many problems only made me sad, and increased my determination to get better and get out of there.

Chapter 12
THE ROLES OF THE PSYCHOLOGICAL & RECREATIONAL THERAPISTS

After a few weeks, I realized that being in the rehab hospital was doing me a world of good, but being surrounded by sick people and the growing awareness of my own disabilities caused me to become quite depressed. I tried attending a couple of discussion groups organized by Psychological Services, but after sitting for an hour hearing other patients talk about how their stroke occurred and how it made them feel, I only left more depressed.

To me, recreation therapy involved reading the newspaper, having a cigarette, and taking a nap, but the staff didn't seem to buy into my program.

So, to my schedule of physical, occupational and speech therapy were added a couple of sessions of **psychological therapy.**

I guess there was some small comfort in being able to talk

confidentially with a trained counselor, however it wasn't long before I felt like that was going nowhere, too. Yes, I had a stroke. Yes, I am depressed. Yes, I have a lot to be thankful for. But unfortunately it never went any further than that, and my therapist neglected to tell me that there was also a psychiatrist on staff who might have at least prescribed some medication to keep me out of the dumps. It wasn't until months after I was released from rehab that I found some relief by meeting regularly with a talented counselor and a psychiatrist who shared a practice near our home.

Recreational therapy was also offered at the hospital. I'm pretty much a loner, and never cared for getting up a group for chess, checkers or cards. The rest of the activities they offered—sewing, calligraphy and basket weaving—were definitely not my cup of tea. To me, recreation was reading the newspaper, having a cigarette, and taking a nap, but the staff didn't seem to buy into my program.

We did agree on one activity—baking homemade bread. My wife brought in our bread machine, and once a week the recreation therapy corridor was filled with the smells of cheese, multigrain, and a hearty white bread. The work helped me feel like my old self again, and sharing the fruits of our labor made the staff and patients feel pretty good, too.

One Friday, I heard that the Rec staff was hosting a "Happy Hour." Having the greatest respect for a well-made cocktail, I made a beeline for the main lounge. Imagine my disappointment when I discovered there were lots of little snacks, but no drinks. Another disappointment, but another good reason to hurry up and get better so I could get out of there!

STROKE

Chapter 13
TWO STEPS FORWARD, ONE STEP BACK

All told, I stayed at the rehab hospital for three-and-a-half months. There were good days and bad days—times I could tell I was improving and times I felt I would never get any better. Although I knew staying at the facility was the best thing for me, there were many sleepless nights when I lay awake and considered just giving up. In fact, for several nights I actually plotted how I might escape the place and just run away.

There was one really bright young man at the facility who, prior to sustaining a serious brain injury, had been a successful teacher and before his accident was planning on doing further graduate work at

All told, I stayed at the rehab hospital for three-and-a-half months. There were good days and bad days—times I could tell I was improving and times I felt I would never get any better.

an Ivy League school. One night there was a great commotion and I learned the next day that he had gotten fed up with the regimentation of institutional life and simply walked out of the facility. I never heard the details, but apparently the hospital staff notified the police who called his parents and within hours he was back in his room. I figured that if a guy his age with the use of both legs couldn't get away, there was little hope my plot would succeed. There was one other patient who obviously had plans to go on the lam. Each day he would get up and pack his bags and go sit on his suitcase outside of the door of his room. No one ever came to pick him up, and one day I noticed he was no longer there. I never found out what happened to him.

I guess one thing that made life at the rehab hospital so difficult was the loss of control over your own life. You couldn't get up when you wanted to, or make a snack when you were hungry, or go outside unassisted. Everything was by the book… routine… like being back in the Army. There was never any privacy—you were always part of a group of similarly broken down and disaffected people. And even though I was a professional trained to work with the handicapped, I had very little say about my own therapeutic program. They had a system, they had a schedule, and it was "their way or the highway." There were many days when, as hard as I worked, I didn't see any progress and I would go back to my room and wonder if I would ever get any better. The depression, monotony and despair were really starting to take their toll.

One day I received a package from an old friend. Inside

was a book by Dr. Robert Schuller, the well-known author and minister from Southern California's Crystal Cathedral. The friend, who I had known since the 1950s when she was my son's third grade teacher, wrote a thoughtful note inside, but it was the book's title that brought me to tears—*Tough Times Don't Last, Tough People Do.* I made a resolution that day—one that I have had to renew many times since—that I would hang in there and keep working, keep hoping, keep believing.

Shortly thereafter, my perseverance was rewarded with a weekend pass. Although the doctors didn't think I was ready to go home for good, they felt it would be a worthwhile experience to let me spend a couple of days in my old surroundings. I think I had mixed emotions. Would it be the same? How would the neighbors react to seeing me half-crippled and in a wheelchair? Would I like it so much that I wouldn't want to go back to rehab?

There were also a few practical matters. Were my legs strong enough that I would be able to climb up into our Jeep? Was there room in the condo for me to move around in my wheelchair? What about all the medication I was taking—would Eleanor and I be able to administer it correctly at home? And what if something happened? What if I fell or had another stroke? As much as I wanted to get out of there, it made me nervous to be away from the physicians and therapists and assistants who had become such a part of my routine.

My son and his wife, who since the stroke were making plans to move nearby, were in town for the weekend. My daughter and her husband lived just a few miles away, so between all of us we worked together and pulled it off. I was glad to see my dog, the view of the ocean we enjoy from our balcony, and share a few meals at home with my family. I must confess, I also really enjoyed sleeping in my own bed again, and spent not a little bit of time snoozing. The family helped get me back to the rehab hospital on time, and the adventure was judged by all to have been a success.

It was another five weeks before I was actually released from the hospital for good. During that period my time was spent learning new ways to do old activities, increasing my physical endurance, and of course, learning to cope with my limitations and the attendant pain. When the doctors finally announced that they thought I was ready to go home for good, I was out of there as fast as I could pack my bags. I had spent nearly 100 nights in that place—away from home, away from family—and 100 days alternately worrying, working, complaining and praying. Two steps forward— one step back. And now one giant step on the road to recovery.

I spent nearly 100 nights in that rehab hospital—away from home, away from family—and 100 days alternately worrying, working, complaining and praying. Two steps forward—one step back. And now one giant step on the road to recovery.

Chapter 14
MAKING THE HOUSE MORE ACCESSIBLE

I think my wife was as excited about my being released from the rehab hospital as I was. Weeks before my homecoming, she began preparing our condo for my return.

Thankfully, our building was relatively new, and therefore met all of the current standards for being "barrier-free" and "handicapped accessible." Since 1991, with the passing of the Americans with Disabilities Act, all newly-constructed buildings have to meet certain federal standards for accessibility. Typically that means reserved parking spaces near the entrance for

Since 1991, with the passing of the Americans with Disabilities Act, all newly-constructed buildings have to meet certain federal standards for accessibility.

handicapped drivers, walkways and hallways of sufficient width to accommodate wheelchairs, and ramps, lifts or elevators as an alternative to stairs. Getting into our building was easy, but we soon came to find out that the laws only govern the design of common areas, not the individual condominium units. Months after my arrival back home, we were still making adjustments inside our condo to make getting around easier.

To help us sort through what we could do to make the place more suited to my special needs, my physical and occupational therapists agreed to come over to go through the apartment with us. Right away they had a number of helpful suggestions. They had us remove all small rugs that might slip under one's feet, and reposition any furniture on which one could trip or that might be in the way of the wheelchair. They urged us to tape or tack down all larger carpets, and to remove any electrical cords that were not up against the wall. For the bathroom, they suggested a bath bench and a raised toilet seat to make transfers easier, and in the bedroom they had some very helpful suggestions about how to rearrange the furniture to make it easier for me to access the bed, my dresser and the closet.

One of the first things my wife did was to buy one of those adjustable beds like the one to which I had become accustomed in the hospital. Not only are they more comfortable than most normal beds, their adjustability makes transferring from the bed to the wheelchair or to a standing position much easier and safer. We were able to set up two electric twin beds side-by-side so that we could both adjust them to suit our preferences, and we added side rails to mine to give me something to grab on to during transfers or when I wanted to turn over. Even before the stroke, I had a fondness for spending lots of lazy hours reading or watching the television in bed, so I figured that whatever time and money we put into getting this right was well worth it.

Our daughter, Nancy, hunted until she found a bedside table on wheels, much like the over-the-bed tables found in hospitals. There I can keep water, pills, tissues, reading materials, a lamp, the telephone, an alarm clock and the occasional bedtime snack—all near at hand so that I don't have to bother my wife in the middle of the night.

Home Accessibility Checklist
- [ ] *Rearrange the furniture*
- [ ] *Install grab bars*
- [ ] *Remove all small rugs*
- [ ] *Tape down larger rugs*
- [ ] *Move electrical wires*
- [ ] *Get a bath bench*
- [ ] *Install a raised toilet seat*
- [ ] *Consider an adjustable bed and an electric reclining chair*
- [ ] *Reorganize shelves*
- [ ] *Get a mechanical reacher*
- [ ] *Get a wireless intercom for room-to-room communication*

Next we turned our attention to the bathroom. I'll confess that the bathroom has always been one of the most important rooms in our house. Where else can you completely get away from the phone and other people and have a little privacy? Give me the daily newspaper, a stack of magazines, and maybe a cup of coffee, and I can stay in there for hours. But in our condo, the bathroom door wasn't even wide enough for me to get through in my wheelchair. Off came the door. Up came the bath rugs. Out went the linen cabinet. I was determined to preserve my "reading room."

There were numerous adjustments to follow. For starters, your typical toilet is quite low to the ground, making transfers all the more difficult—and dangerous. The first thing we did was buy a raised toilet seat like we had seen at the rehab hospital. The local medical supply house had a number of good options, including an aluminum over-the-toilet chair comprised of a light-weight but rigid frame with arms to help in transfers. With a nifty insert, this chair could also be used at bedside, or even folded up and taken on trips. While we're on the subject, I've also been grateful numerous times that we keep a urinal beside the bed and have a waterproof mattress pad for those times when you just can't get to the bathroom fast enough.

When it comes to bathing, I've always preferred a shower to a tub bath. Unfortunately, our shower stall had a narrow doorway, made all the more difficult by a four-inch-high threshold over which I wasn't able to lift my leg. The therapists had suggested using the tub with a bath bench, a four-legged plastic bench that you set up with two legs on the bathroom floor and two legs in the tub. The idea is to sit on the bench and then slide across it into the tub. The problem is you have to have someone help you swing your legs in and out of the tub, at great cost to your modesty. I balked! I was determined to figure out how to use the shower. Finally, someone came up with the idea of replacing the glass shower door and its frame with a shower curtain, thus widening the entryway by several inches. A handyman was called in to lower the four-inch threshold so that I could more easily walk in. Once in the shower, the bath bench allowed me to sit while washing, and several strategically-placed grab bars made it a much safer and enjoyable experience. "One giant step for mankind!"

Other bathroom tricks we had to learn included using two non-slip bath mats—one inside and one outside the shower stall to avoid slipping on wet tile. A shampoo dispenser with suction cups was attached to the wall so that I could use it with one hand. Soap-on-a-rope, a long-handled brush and a handheld shower head made the whole process much easier. Over at the sink, we arranged all of my toiletries on the counter so that I could easily reach them, lowered the towel bar to wheelchair-height, and installed a magnified extension mirror for shaving and "primping."

Down the hall was the next most important room—the kitchen. I've always enjoyed cooking and baking, not to mention tending bar for family and friends. Whoever thought up the "galley kitchen"—those long, narrow work areas where everything is supposedly within reach— sure wasn't thinking about people in wheelchairs. And you should see the dance my wife and I have to do when we both want to be in there at the same time. I don't think we'll really be happy with it until we can totally redesign the kitchen, but we have been able to make a few adjustments that help out. Thankfully, we already had a side-by-side refrigerator with an ice maker and water dispenser on the door. And the pantry has accordion-style folding doors that are much easier to use than a full-sized door that swings in such a wide arc. Eleanor was willing to rearrange the cupboards so that the items that I use most often were kept on the lower shelves, and a faucet with a long lever allows me to use the kitchen sink. Other important pointers for using the kitchen include having a stove that has the controls on the front so you don't have to reach across hot burners to change the temperature. Several companies make kitchen accessories that are designed for one-handed use, such as pepper grinders, jar openers, and cutting boards that hold items in place for slicing. We've found a couple of "reachers" that come in handy for getting to things that are too high or in the back of the cupboard. Ideally, the perfect wheelchair-accessible kitchen would have plenty of floor space, lower counters, and roll-under appliances—like cook tops and sinks with leg room underneath instead of cabinets. But if you're willing to take a little more time and be a little more conscious of safety concerns, even a small kitchen can be made more functional.

Although I'm retired, we realized I needed a desk where I could go through the mail, write letters and such. In a one-handed world, you need a large, uncluttered work surface to get anything done, so we had a desk custom made that was the right height and width for my wheelchair. For relaxing, we bought one of those electric reclining chairs which, like our bed, can be moved into a variety of positions with the push of a button. Raised into the up position, I can more easily transfer to the chair from a standing position. A pocket on the side of the chair holds the controls and the TV remote.

Since rehabilitation is an ongoing process, we had a grab bar installed in the den so that I can periodically stand and do exercises. It also provides a welcome relief from "fanny fatigue."

Gardening is one of my hobbies, but getting outside is difficult, so my wife set up a miniature greenhouse in the den that holds a dozen or so orchids and African violets. That way I can just roll to the kitchen, fill up the watering pot, and tend my mini-garden at my leisure.

Since our kitchen is so small, we typically take our meals in the dining room. Before the stroke, I never could have imagined how many tables in homes and most restaurants are so low that you can't get under them in a wheelchair without skinning your knees. Once again, we were fortunate to be able to have a table made to accommodate my needs. The height works for both our dining room chairs and my wheel chair, and the pedestal base keeps me from banging up the legs.

Moving from room to room was an issue we had to confront. Three-fourths of our apartment had wall-to-wall carpeting—beautiful to look at, but the deep pile made maneuvering a wheelchair very difficult. After much research, we decided to replace the carpet with tile. Wood or linoleum would have achieved the same effect. Now both walking and using the chair are easier. We also added clear plastic protectors on the edges of any walls that were susceptible to getting nicked if I cut the corners too sharply.

In the course of making the home more accessible, we

came across a number of appliances and aids that proved helpful. I'm one of those people who would be happier if Alexander Graham Bell had never invented the telephone, but I do appreciate the cordless phone my son got for us. I can use it at my desk, in my recliner, or simply keep it in the wheelchair so that it's always with me. The speed dial feature makes calling my wife's cell phone, the neighbors, the doctor or our children a snap, since I don't have to remember the numbers or push a long series of buttons. We also make good use of an old wireless intercom system that was originally bought for our granddaughter. We have one unit set up by my bedside, another in the den, another in the kitchen and one in the spare bedroom where my wife has a desk. That intercom has come in handy more than a few times when I needed to call for help and Eleanor was in some other part of the house.

My daughter-in-law gave me a large-number clock with time and date, and my son set up our computer so that the screen is easier to read. I even got some of that voice-activated software that supposedly lets you dictate your thoughts to the computer and it types the words out for you, but so far it and I are not communicating too well. Two other gadgets that we've considered getting are sound-activated light switches ("Clap-on, clap-off") and an emergency alert device that when activated, dials directly to the hospital and sends a request for help.

We've listed a number of good sources for assistive devices and accessible living ideas in the final section, "Stroke Resources." Ask your doctor and rehabilitation therapists for solutions to whatever problems you may face at home.

Chapter 15
OUTPATIENT THERAPY & HOME HEALTH CARE

After getting things settled at home, it was time to resume my therapies, this time as an **outpatient.** Instead of living in the rehab facility, it was arranged that I would go back several days a week to continue my therapy. However, I soon found out that even though it was the same facility, being an outpatient meant dealing with new staff, new therapists, and new ways of doing things.

Going to therapy no longer involved just rolling down the hall. The actual work was preceded by about two hours of "warm-up exercises." Getting up, dressing, eating, taking pills, making my way down the hall and into the car, and then, once we had completed the 25-minute drive, transferring out of the car, getting inside and registering each day. With all that preparation, the actual therapy session and the return trip home, I got about four hours of exercise for every one hour of therapy.

Since walking was still my priority, the first appointment of the day was always PT. The physical therapist I worked with when I was an inpatient was very good with me, and she went the extra mile to recommend to the outpatient office that I get to work with a friend of hers whom she thought was the best. We, too, hit it off, and the hard work of the sessions was interspersed with all manner of humor, wisecracks and taunts. I would tease her about her life as a single woman, and she would goad me about my laziness and inclination to avoid hard work. Over the next year, she and I worked together

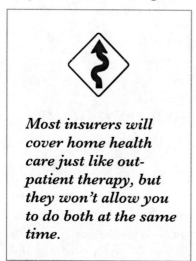

Most insurers will cover home health care just like outpatient therapy, but they won't allow you to do both at the same time.

long enough that I saw her get engaged, married and pregnant, and she helped me progress in my walking to the extent that I could move along at a pretty good pace, and my gait developed a smoothness and naturalness that we hadn't thought possible.

Not all of my outpatient therapy was so rewarding. OT still seemed like a complete waste of time with its childish activities. But we were able to redeem the time with range of motion exercises to keep me limber and heat treatments to ease the shoulder pain that still plagued me.

After commuting to therapy for a while, Eleanor and I both began to tire of the process. It seemed like every waking moment was taken up with getting ready and getting to therapy. I was exhausted, and she never had any time to get anything else done. After a meeting with my outpatient case manager, we decided to take a week off and then resume treatment on a home health care basis.

Home health care provided a wonderful alternative. Several days of research turned up a handful of providers with which our insurance would work. (Most insurers will cover home health care just like outpatient therapy, but they won't allow you to do both at the same time.) Eleanor was diligent to call all of them and assess their services. Once we settled on a company that sounded good, they sent over a case manager to do an initial evaluation of my needs. A full service home health care company can provide a myriad of services—assistance with bathing, dressing and eating, basic medical services like checking your temperature and blood pressure, as well as administering medications, and even basic meal preparation. They also can provide in-home physical, occupational and speech therapists.

The good news about home health care is that all of the service personnel come to you. The bad news is that your house becomes like Grand Central station as half a dozen different people come in and out every day—that is, if they come at all. Most of the home health people we worked with were dear souls, but as independent service providers, they lead complicated lives, driving all over the county to see a wide range of patients during any given day. Inevitably, they (and sometimes, we) would fall behind schedule and need to make alternate plans. Eleanor traded in her exhaustion as a taxi cab driver for the tedium of being a human resources manager and traffic cop.

I remember one week that was particularly unbearable. To our usual schedule of two home health aides, a PT, OT and ST, were added a workman widening the kitchen doorway so that my chair would fit through, a contractor taking measurements to replace our wall-to-wall carpeting with ceramic tile to make the condo easier to maneuver, a helpful neighbor dropping off a lasagna for any easy meal, and amidst all this, the air conditioner for the entire building was being serviced. All day the phone rang, the doorbell buzzed, and the revolving door kept swinging— all in the 90-degree heat of a hot Florida day! Over dinner that night we decided that this pace was not therapeutic for Eleanor or me, so we canceled all services for the next couple of days and took a long weekend off.

Over the past few years, we've alternated between outpatient therapy, home health care and periodic "vacations." Each approach has its benefits, and we found that we were most happy with a mix of all three.

Chapter 16
PUBLIC ACCESSIBILITY

Speaking of vacations, a brief word about the state of public accessibility. Since the federal government passed the Americans with Disabilities Act, most public places have done at least the bare minimum to comply with their guidelines. But I must say that seldom do I leave the house that I don't run into some kind of accessibility problem. Before I became disabled, handicapped parking spaces seemed to be everywhere. Now that I need them, they are invariably full. When there are available spaces, you often end up having to go way out of your way before you can find a cut through the curb to roll up to the sidewalk. I can't count the times I've wished there had been some sort of cover over the parking lot. Ever try to get out of car and into your wheelchair in the midst of a downpour? Both your chair and you end up getting soaked—not the way you want to start a long day of errands or begin a nice evening at a restaurant.

Speaking of restaurants, most could do a significantly better job for their handicapped clients. How many times must I hear, "Would you like to wait in the bar while we prepare your table?" No thanks. Have you ever tried to get the attention of a bartender when he can't even see your head above the counter? "Would you like a booth?" Well, no. Since the table tops of most booths don't hang over the end where you could most easily roll up in a wheelchair, you're guaranteed to leave the restaurant with half of your dinner in your lap. And how about the way most places pack the tables in so tightly that when the hostess says, "Follow me," half the patrons have to rise or move their chairs for you to get by. Nothing like a dramatic entrance into a fine dining establishment to start your night off right.

My (former) favorite restaurant can be called "barrier-free" and "handicapped-accessible" in only the loosest sense of the words. They offer one handicapped parking space which requires you to use a decrepit, pockmarked ramp that leads to a narrow sidewalk riddled with more cracks than the San Andreas Fault. I arrived one night to find a lady laying prostate, bleeding from the head, having taken a bad spill at the main entrance. Although my wife and I both have spoken to the manager and the hostess several times, they just keep repeating that their facility meets all federal standards.... Right.

Fast food and family restaurants present their own set of challenges. Ever try to open one of those butter pats wrapped in gold foil with just one hand? What with straws, salt and pepper, ketchup and creamers all being packaged in some sort of paper container, it's a wonder you ever get around to eating your meal at all.

When it comes to doors on public buildings, those that automatically open are clearly the most desirable. Oddly, not a one of my doctors or specialists has one. When I go to my dentist, I don't have to wait until I'm inside for the torture to begin. It's always a matter of grappling with a heavy door while trying not to roll backwards down the ramp. Heaven help you if you're carrying something in your lap. When we attend church we're presented with two options: a covered entrance for inclement weather… but it only has stairs; or a ramp so steep that it takes all of my wife's strength to get me up to the door. When we exit on the ramp, we have to ask an usher to hold the wheelchair back so that I don't go flying down the slope and out into the parking lot.

Those electric shopping carts that you see at the front of most grocery stores make a nice statement— "Handicapped people welcome." But try driving one through overstocked aisles complete with cardboard displays of the latest special. "Clean up on aisle nine!"

Although most public places now provide handicapped-accessible bathrooms, what that means varies wildly. A cramped toilet stall with illogically-placed grab bars is usually what you get. And if you're able to maneuver your way in, don't expect to be able to reach the soap or paper towels. I don't mean to be complaining, but it only takes a couple of bad experiences to make you want to call out the dogs, if not the attorneys.

One encouraging trend is the appearance of more family and unisex restrooms, typically marked by both a men's and women's restroom symbol. The majority of these rooms are spacious and yet private, allowing a spouse to assist a mate of the opposite sex without embarrassment.

Care to take in a movie? Better get there early. While many theaters provide space for wheelchairs at the end of selected aisles, they're usually way down front or up in the nosebleed section. Need cash? ATMs are generally placed at the right height for wheelchair use, but if the machine is enclosed in a small "secure" area, better plan on having someone else go for the gold. By the time you get in and out, all the stores will be closed and you'll go home empty-handed. I've found only one store at our mall that has placed a counter low enough for wheelchair patrons to write a check or sign a credit card slip. Believe me, they get my business every birthday, anniversary and Christmas.

Travel, since 9/11, has gotten more difficult for everyone, but imagine taking a trip from a wheelchair. We normally take a shuttle van to the airport to avoid the trek from the long-term parking lot. That means a difficult transfer from the wheelchair up into the van and then back to the wheelchair. Once inside the airport, things usually go smoothly at the ticket counter, and even security hasn't been too bad. But the minute you try to board the plane, things take a turn for the worse. Typically you are asked to transfer from your personal wheelchair to an exceedingly narrow straight-backed wheelchair on which you are unceremoniously carted backwards down the aisle like a sack of potatoes at a farm market. Standing, and trying to slide into the ever-shrinking space between seats, takes time and patience on the part of you, your companion, the flight attendants and your fellow travelers. I propose that it become a mandatory policy that every airline passenger who has to go through this experience be immediately offered an alcoholic beverage of their choice—no charge.

Once at your destination—no matter how much it has been advertised as a vacation paradise—you're faced with the same obstacles and challenges as back home. Most hotel and motel chains have a few handicapped-accessible rooms to rent. Again, make your plans early. And check to find out if the rooms are handicapped- or wheelchair-accessible. There's a big difference. The designation "handicapped" may mean only that there are grab bars in the bathroom and a broken down bath bench in the tub. A true "wheelchair

There's a big difference between a "handicapped" motel room and one designated as "wheelchair accessible." A true "wheelchair accessible" room will have extra floor space, a large bathroom with a roll-in shower stall and a roll-under sink, and plenty of room to position your wheelchair so that transfers to the toilet, shower and bed are safe.

accessible" room will have extra floor space, a large bathroom with a roll-in shower stall and a roll-under sink, and plenty of room to position your wheelchair so that transfers to the toilet, shower and bed are safe. Handicapped- versus wheelchair-accessible: make the time to make the distinction when you make your hotel reservation. You might actually feel like you're "on vacation."

STROKE

Chapter 17
CAREGIVING
A Word from Eleanor Prillaman

Throughout our lives, we all typically take turns caring for one another. Short-term illnesses, minor injuries and temporary setbacks give us each an opportunity to put aside our own needs and help a friend or family member get through a rough time. When a major debilitating illness strikes, sometimes one person has to carry more than his own load for a long time, and it is this ongoing process of providing help that is meant when people use the term **"caregiving."**

When a major debilitating illness strikes, sometimes one person has to carry more than his own load for a long time, and it is this ongoing process of providing help that is meant when people use the term "caregiving."

In our case, "caregiving" didn't just miraculously start the day Doug came home from the rehabilitation hospital. It began the very moment the brain attack struck—quick, unexpected, and with no warning whatsoever.

When Doug fell the third time, I knew that something very serious was occurring, yet he continued to deny that there was anything wrong. My first job as caregiver was to forgo our usual style of making joint decisions and insist that we go to the hospital. Since our preferred hospital was in the next town, I knew I couldn't call 911 because they would, by law, insist on taking us to the nearest hospital, with which we were not familiar. We agreed that I would call a neighbor and ask them to drive Doug, while I followed in our car.

On the way to the hospital, it began to sink in that my husband was experiencing a potentially serious medical incident. I didn't know exactly what was happening, but it was comforting to have friends go with us to the emergency room. Once he was admitted and I knew I had the support of the medical staff, I urged our friends to return home. As I walked behind the gurney through a maze of hallways, my anxiety level was great, but having them there had been a big help.

As soon as daylight arrived, I called our children to tell them what little I knew at that point: simply, Dad had had a stroke and he was in the hospital. Our daughter and her husband, who lived in a nearby Florida town, arrived almost immediately. Our son and his wife headed south from their home in Virginia. At times such as this, one thanks God for loving, caring children. Their presence was helpful to Doug and of immeasurable benefit to my physical and emotional stability.

Dr. Shafer, the admitting **neurologist** whom I had not yet met, called after examining Doug. Yes, he had indeed experienced a stroke, a right brain attack resulting in damage to the left side of his body. My heart sank. "How much damage?" "How was he affected?" I had so many questions and so much apprehension. Dr. Shafer's replies were general yet alarming. "He's had a major stroke. Time will tell just what faculties have been affected and the extent of the damage."

The image I projected during these early hours was probably one of being in control, but deep inside I felt like my heart was running away. I shared this with my daughter-in-law and at her insistence we had my blood pressure checked. Although I was being successfully treated for high blood pressure, the readings were alarmingly high. For some reason, on a hunch the doctor felt I should have a urinalysis, although I had no symptoms of a problem. Sure enough, the test proved positive, and medication for both a bladder infection and anxiety were prescribed. That incident was the first of many in which I realized that a stroke affects not only the patient, but that the attendant stress can trigger problems for the caregiver as well.

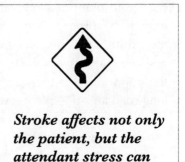

Stroke affects not only the patient, but the attendant stress can trigger problems for the caregiver as well.

I was a little uncomfortable that the admitting doctor had never seen Doug before, but my confidence in his abilities and the skill of the nursing staff grew over the ensuing days. Doug's primary nurse was truly Florence Nightingale incarnate. If she wasn't by his side, she was just outside his door. I learned from her that she had orders from Dr. Shafer to call him the instant she had concerns about any new observations. This made me feel more secure, but frightened as well. It only underscored that those first days were touch and go.

Doug stayed in our local hospital for a total of nine days— five in **critical care,** and four in **progressive care.** Initially, the time was taken up with tests and rest. After they felt like Doug had been stabilized, I had my first chance to observe a rehabilitative therapist working with him. The process began with an evaluation, and then moved into basic exercises. As I watched and listened, I realized that this was the beginning of my education about the importance of therapy as a part of caregiving on the long road ahead to recovery.

When we heard that Doug was ready to "graduate" and move over to the rehabilitation hospital, we were all so elated. However, our happiness quickly turned to frustration when the transition between the two facilities proved to be so poorly planned. No one could tell me when or how Doug would be moved, and as it turned out, no one at the rehab hospital knew when he was arriving or much about his needs. Once again I had to take on a new caretaking role, that of institutional troubleshooter. After much prodding, I was able to find out that the confusion was due to a lack of communication between hospital and rehab facility case managers. It ended up taking the better part of three days to get the mess worked out.

Not only did we change hospitals, but doctors as well. Doug's neurologist referred us to a co-worker, a rehabilitation physiatrist, who would coordinate the treatment for the next three-and-a-half months at the **rehabilitation hospital.** But because she made her daily rounds at 7:30 a.m., long before I could easily get to the hospital, I seldom got to meet with her face-to-face. For the first few weeks, our only communication was with notes left with the head nurse. This lack of contact with the person making most of the decisions was another cause for concern. As a backup, I asked that Doug's regular primary care physician be called for a consult. He responded immediately, and I felt much better when he had given Doug a once over and recommended a slight medication change.

I came to admire most of the nursing staff, especially the aides who, we quickly learn-ed, were the hands-on work horses. Seldom did one come to assist Doug without a smile and an encouraging attitude. I observed the care with which the

As a caregiver, one must balance high expectations with patience, firmness with tender loving care, and understand that sometimes the best medicine is simply a good joke.

medications were administered and recorded. I came to understand that going to the dining rooms for meals, even when the patient didn't prefer to, fostered socialization which was an important part of the rehabilitation process. But mostly I learned that when it comes to being a caregiver, one must balance high expectations with patience, firmness with tender loving care, and that sometimes, the best medicine is simply a good joke.

As often as I could, I visited the hospital during Doug's therapy sessions. It was wonderful to see him working so hard to get better. I'll never forget the day I came in to meet him for dinner and found him sitting up straight in his chair, just as he always had prior to the stroke. Another unforgettable moment was the first time I saw him stand upright during **physical therapy.** It took two trained therapists, one on each side of him to assist, but stand he did, and for the first time since the stroke he put weight on his own two feet. One giant step, indeed.

I also visited regularly so that I could learn how to help Doug continue making progress once he came home. My education began with simply observing how the therapists worked with him, then progressed to conferences, and finally moved in to hands-on training with each specialist.

Much transpired during Doug's three-and-a-half month hospital stay that was helpful to us both—but all was not perfect. Again, the weak thread in the whole tapestry was the **case manager.** Had I not been so actively involved, I don't think Doug would have gotten the attention he needed, and at the same time, I would have known little about his progress. The therapists and the attending physician met on a regular basis to review each patient's progress, but families and patients were not invited to participate in these sessions. We only got information second hand—and that only when we asked for it. At one critical juncture when the decision was being made as to whether Doug should stay in the rehab facility or be discharged, we had to demand a face-to-face meeting with his case manager, and even that proved not very satisfying. Lesson learned: the caregiver has to manage the case manager!

When the decision was made to discharge him, we were all greatly relieved that he would be coming home. In my eagerness to have Doug back, I felt invincible—I was sure I could do it all: administer medications, be his home therapist, provide personal care and moral support... everything! Unfortunately, no one had warned me that the responsibility of a full-time caregiver can become overwhelming, both physically and emotionally. Doug was discharged with a packet of prescriptions for his medications and instructions to see his neurologist and internist in three months. Other than that, we were on our own!

With Doug back at home, my caregiver role changed from that of observer and cheerleader to multifaceted project manager. First, I had to prepare our condo for his safety and comfort, which included buying several pieces of new furniture and rearranging the rooms for greater accessibility. Next I had to learn about various assistive devices that would help him around the house: a raised toilet seat with arms; grab bars in the bathroom and other strategic locations; a mechanical "reacher" to help him get things one couldn't normally access from a sitting position. Then there was the demolition of walls and the widening of doorways for the wheelchair to fit through.

Although Doug was out of the hospital, his therapy was to be ongoing. We had been told that we could pursue either in-home or outpatient therapy, but no one had really explained to us the pros and cons of either. Since we were already familiar with the rehab facility, Doug opted to go back to the hospital several times a week as an **outpatient.** After making our decision, we were told to wait for a call from the scheduling office.

A big part of caregiving is being the squeaky wheel.

Ten days passed and still, no call. We were both getting anxious because Doug had worked hard during his hospital stay and we didn't want him to lose his new skills. Plus, he had developed constant post-stroke left arm pain and he desperately needed both therapy and medication. It took a call to our former attending physician at the hospital to get help. She was as upset as I that the transition to outpatient status had taken so long. She immediately ordered pain medication and arranged for Doug to receive therapy at home while we waited for the outpatient service to get their act together. Part of caregiving is being the squeaky wheel.

Speaking of wheels, being an outpatient means you spend a lot of time on the road. I had heard that the hospital offered van pick-up services for patients, but on further inquiry was told that we did not qualify since we lived in an adjacent county. Subsequent calls to the local Social Services department, the Council on Aging and AARP all yielded the same results—they offered transportation services, but regulations would not permit them to transport patients from one jurisdiction to another. So, between my son, daughter and myself, we shared chauffeur duties, leaving home at 8:30 in the morning and returning later that afternoon.

Although we were grateful that Doug was continuing to make progress, out-patient care was very difficult for both of us. The long hours and great physical demands, along with Doug's continuing post-stroke pain and some medication side effects, began taking their toll. After careful consideration, it was decided that Home Health services would better meet his needs.

Caregiving Checklist
- [ ] *Prepare the home*
- [ ] *Manage medications*
- [ ] *Help with exercises*
- [ ] *Coordinate home health care workers*
- [ ] *Manage insurance claims*
- [ ] *Keep a schedule of follow-up appointments*
- [ ] *Pace yourself, and ask for help*
- [ ] *Take regular breaks for your own physical and emotional well-being*

We did have some concerns that home health therapists might be less qualified than those at the hospital, but our fears were groundless. We soon learned that one hour of one-on-one therapy three times per week with these talented professionals could be more productive than five one-hour sessions with other patients being treated in the same room. Plus, it made a lot of sense for the therapists to work with Doug in his own home environment—walking in and around our condo, learning how to safely use his shower, getting out onto the balcony to enjoy the view.... The home environment also proved to be a perfect place for the speech therapist to stretch his cognitive and reading comprehension skills, as well as to help him continue learning how to compensate for his left neglect. The occupational therapist was wonderful—helping him gauge how to manipulate his wheelchair throughout our home without running into walls and furniture. It may sound minor, but I will never forget the first time Doug was able to wheel himself throughout the house as needed without my help. Not only did it mean more independence for him, but more free time for me!

I should mention that since many stroke survivors end up spending a considerable amount of time in their wheelchairs, choosing one that is the right size and design is very important. Wheelchairs come in several styles, based on the patient's needs and body type, as well as how you plan to use it. The chair's stability, durability, weight and maneuverability are all important factors. Perhaps the first decision is what sort of propulsion you want—hand, foot or motorized. If you choose a motorized chair, do you want the scooter style, or a true power wheelchair? Do you want a rigid chair, which feels more solid on the ground, or a folding chair which is easier to move in and out of the car? Do you want handles on the back that will make it easier for the caregiver to push? Then there are the decisions about wheels (large or small) and tires (hard rubber or air-filled).

Once you've chosen the basic elements, there are all manner of adjustments to be made. Your loved one's height and weight will dictate the seat width, depth and height, but the armrests, footrests and backrest all need to be adjusted for maximum performance. Some people think that they can just use any old hand-me-down wheelchair; after all, "it was good enough for Grandma." But the match of user to wheelchair is like a good marriage, and should be officiated by experienced therapists or other trained professionals. The good news is, if your doctor writes a prescription for the chair, there's a very good chance that Medicare or Medicaid will pay for it.

The match of user to wheelchair is like a good marriage, and should be officiated by experienced therapists or other trained professionals.

Once we selected the right chair, the first accessory we added was a specially-designed seat cushion that provides both comfort and protection from chair sores. Next, I bought a backpack that we hung on the back of the chair. In its several zippered compartments Doug can carry his wallet, keys, sunglasses, magazines, medication, and even a urinal and change of clothes in case he has an accident while away from home. A third helpful feature we added was a lumbar-support pillow for his back.

Since a wheelchair is such an important part of Doug's mobility, it was worth it to learn all we could about making it a safe and comfortable ride. Once we had an appropriate chair, the therapists worked with Doug on how to safely transfer from the wheelchair to the bed, his recliner, or the toilet.

Even with all our best planning, accidents do happen. Although I normally assisted Doug whenever he needed to go to the bathroom, one day he decided not to bother me and headed down the hall without letting me know. I heard a frantic call—"Eleanor! Eleanor!"—and then a loud crash. I ran to the bathroom to find him on the floor—the back of his head up against the shower and his feet tangled in the wheels of the chair which had toppled over on its side. I was able to extricate his feet and move him into a prone position, putting a pillow under his head and covering him with a blanket. I then called 911 and asked for the EMTs to come help him up and check him over to see if he needed to go to the emergency room. Their response was prompt and efficient, and there were no signs that the fall was the result of anything other than a mishap. Doug's heart rate, oxygen level, temperature and blood sugar were all in the normal range. He had a few minor scrapes on his leg and ankle, but the evaluation did not indicate that he needed further medical attention. He complained of some chest discomfort around the rib cage, for which the EMTs gave him Tylenol, and we helped him into his favorite recliner to relax before dinner. It ended up being a relatively small incident, but it served as a good reminder that both patient and caregiver alike need to find a balance between independence and caution.

Medication management was a full-time job for the nurses at the rehab facility, and, once the patient comes home, it can be a full-time job for the caregiver.

To guard against any further problem with blood clotting, Doug was taking various blood thinners such as Ticlid™, Plavix™ and good old aspirin. Capoten™ helps him control blood pressure.

Medication management can be a full-time job for the caregiver. Keeping a myriad of prescriptions straight can be a daunting task.

Since the stroke paralyzed or weakened the muscles on one side of his body, it's natural that it affected his bladder control also. To help completely empty the bladder, he takes Flomax™, and to combat urgent and frequent urination, he's taken Ditropan™ and Pyridium Plus™.
For depression, I think Doug has tried every drug ever invented, including Effexor™, Celexa™, Zoloft™, Zerzone™, Prozac™ and Wellbutrin™, which come to find out has the same active ingredients as Zyban™, the pill he was taking just before the stroke to try to stop smoking. For anxiety, he's used Elavil™ and Buspar™, and if the stroke makes him confused about time and

place and people, he's tried Risperdal™, Zyprexa™ and Seroquil™.

For pain, depending on its severity, he takes either Tylenol™, Darvocet™, Lorcet™, or Neurontin™ (a medication normally used as an anti-seizure medication but that also works for chronic pain). For leg cramps, which he's had on-and-off for years due to varicose veins, he takes quinine sulfite.

Between the pain and the depression, Doug often has trouble sleeping—which means the caregiver has trouble sleeping, too. In an effort to find the right pill that worked with the least side affects we tried ProSom™, Ambien™, Dalmane™, mild doses of Valium™, and even Xanax™ when we thought his sleep deprivation might be anxiety-based.

Naturally enough, with all these different drugs coursing through his body, he sometimes got nauseous, which required another pill, Compazine™. Since Doug loves to eat, a daily AcipHex™ comes in handy to keep down the acid reflux, and Lipitor™ or Zocor™ help him keep an eye on his cholesterol. Type 2 diabetes runs in his family, and sure enough he got it, so for that he takes Avandia™, and since he battles chronic bronchitis, we keep an Atrovent™ or Alburetra™ puffer, as well as some Prednisone™, on hand.

Keeping all of this medicine straight can be a daunting task! Two tools have proved invaluable. First, when the doctor prescribes a certain course of medication, I add it to our ongoing list of what Doug is taking. I keep the list on our computer, and leave printouts in the bathroom, in the kitchen, and in my purse, as well as send copies to both of our children. Second, I'm a firm believer in those little pill boxes that have various compartments for each day of the week and several time periods throughout the day. Once a week I organize all of Doug's pills, and then I don't have to worry about it for seven more days.

Have you noticed how, even when the stock market is unpredictable, pharmaceutical stocks show steady growth? It's our family. We take complete credit for keeping scores of biotech companies solvent.

There are a few other handy tools I should mention. Although our main calendar of therapist and doctor appointments is posted on the refrigerator, I also keep a pocket calendar with me at all times. When you're out driving around town, it's hard to envision all of the events crowded on your calendar without your pocket pal. A portable calendar can help you avoid either forgetting about or scheduling conflicting appointments.

I also keep a good supply of underpads at home and in the car. Since transferring from the wheelchair to the toilet can't always happen as quickly as it needs to, these absorbent pads, available at any good drugstore or medical supply house, can really come in handy. I also found a wonderful waterproof mattress pad that is flannel on one side and doesn't make noise or cause sweating like most plastic sheets.

Keep in mind that, even after your loved one is out of the hospital, there will still be follow-up doctor visits and periodic checkups. We routinely see Doug's primary care physician and neurologist, and regularly go to a podiatrist for diabetic foot care, as well as a cardiologist, urologist and ophthalmologist. Together, they keep a watchful eye on Doug's health, and update any prescriptions as needed.

From time to time, the patient may need a "refresher course" in some of the skills initially developed in physical or occupational therapy. Any of the attending physicians may arrange for more intensive therapy via either outpatient or home health care. Once, when we observed that a protracted illness had caused Doug to slip considerably, we arranged for him to be re-admitted as an inpatient at the rehab hospital. This brief "tune up" was just what he needed, and it gave me a break from the daily routine at home.

All of these appointments and prescriptions come at a cost, of course, which adds up to a pile of paperwork. Thankfully, we have Medicare and a supplemental policy which cover most expenses, but there are still so many different forms to file that even a slight mistake can result in enormous costs and the attendant frustration. Our daughter helped us devise a system of tracking all of our medical expenses, and recently has taken over the management of the whole process, for which I am very grateful. That's one hat I don't have to wear in my ever-changing wardrobe as caregiver.

Amidst all of the varied duties involved in continuing care, I simply did not have the time or energy to keep up with the routine housework. Fortunately, we were able to arrange for a lovely lady to become our housekeeper, which freed me of most day-to-day household responsibilities except meal planning and preparation.

One of the most difficult parts of caregiving is to learn when it's time to stop "giving" and take care of yourself. One day, at my husband's insistence, I took a break and went down to the beach with a good book. An hour of lounging at the ocean and walking in the surf was a dose of good medicine for my attitude, patience and mood. And yet it's so hard for me to do, because I always worry that something might happen while I'm away. If an accident occurred, I would feel so guilty.

One of the most difficult parts of caregiving is to learn when it's time to stop "giving" and take care of yourself. If you're mentally and physically exhausted, you won't be of much help.

In the years since Doug's stroke, so much has happened. Our plans to enjoy a lazy life in retirement have changed, and it seems our pace is even busier than it was back when we both worked. There have been times of illness and improved health, fatigue and a resurgence of energy, anguish and joy. Through it all, the one lesson I'm still trying to learn is that I don't have to—and shouldn't—be and do everything for my beloved husband. He needs to have time and space to be by himself. He needs to make his own decisions and retain control of his life. At the same time, I have to think about my own needs as well as his. I need to take breaks, and let other family and friends carry the load for a while. If I'm mentally and physically exhausted, how can I be of any help to him?

I think respecting your own limits is the hardest part of being a loving caregiver. If I can learn this lesson, I know I will have more energy, more patience, more kindness, and more love. Most importantly, I will be a better caregiver, and a better wife.

Respecting your own limits is the hardest part of being a loving caregiver. If I can learn this lesson, I know I will have more energy, more patience, more kindness, and more love. Most importantly, I will be a better caregiver, and a better wife.

Chapter 18
CONTINUED THERAPIES AT HOME

During the months that I worked with a home physical therapist, I mainly continued to focus on improving my walking. Luckily we had a long, carpeted hallway right outside our front door, and that became my "practice field." One of the oddest effects of the kind of stroke I had is that even though you've spent all of your life putting one foot in front of the other, in my case it often took a therapist reminding me how to walk for me to be able to get started. The therapist would give me a cue, saying,

It is one of the prevailing oddities of life after a stroke to realize that there's nothing wrong with your leg—it's just that the message from your brain to the leg is not getting through.

for example, "move your left foot forward," and then I would tell myself "move your left foot forward," and initially at least, nothing would happen. It is one of the prevailing oddities of life after a stroke to realize that there's nothing wrong with, say, your leg—it's just that the message from your brain to the leg is not getting through.

I've read that, at least in the early part of recovery, one of the reasons for repeatedly attempting the same action—even if it's not working—is that your brain may be able to find ways to "re-route" the message "move your leg" so that it goes around the parts of your brain that were damaged and finds a new path to send the signal to your leg. But I've got to tell you, I spent many an hour telling my left leg to move and having nothing happen.

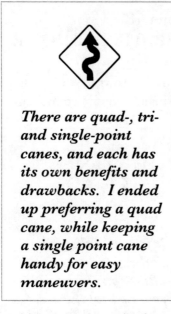

There are quad-, tri- and single-point canes, and each has its own benefits and drawbacks. I ended up preferring a quad cane, while keeping a single point cane handy for easy maneuvers.

Eventually, the therapist decided that we should try a new approach. One was the simple but ingenious tactic of teaching me to lean all of my weight on my right leg and a cane held in my right hand—and to use gravity to cause my nearly-airborne left leg to swing forward. As my wife's father used to say, "there's more than one way to skin a cat," and at least this technique allowed me to get my left foot out in front of the other.

The next step involves the rather frightening prospect of trusting that left leg to hold you up, and supporting all of your weight with the left, and the cane. Even though it only takes a moment to suspend yourself and take a step forward with your right leg, you have the constant fear that you might go crashing to the ground.

We also experimented using different canes. There are quad-, tri- and single-point canes, and each has its own benefits and drawbacks. I ended up preferring a quad cane, while keeping a single point cane handy for easy maneuvers.

While working with the in-home physical therapist, we also experimented with different cues. He originally gave me a four-count cue: cane, tuck, left, right. In order for me to develop a smoother gait, we sometimes used a three-count cue: cane, left, right; and on ambitious days we even experimented with a two-count cue: cane (and left foot), right. When I'm in top shape, the two-count allows me to cover the most ground, but most of the time I'm satisfied to stroll along using the three-count cue. At all speeds, the first priority was safety—not attempting to go it alone without someone walking alongside—and the second was building up my strength, endurance and speed.

The home PT also had me practice walking on different surfaces. Walking on hardwood or tile is relatively easy, but traversing thick carpet or uneven surfaces requires greater care. He also took me outside and had me practice walking on the grass, loose dirt and sand. All required greater concentration and somewhat different approaches.

Since we lived on the sixth floor of a high-rise condo, I had to develop a couple of methods for getting to the ground floor in case of emergency. The first task was to learn how to walk or roll my wheelchair into the elevator without getting rammed by the door. After we mastered that, I began practicing using the stairs. We found that going up and down a relatively short flight of four or five steps was no problem, but, even on the best days, there was no way I was going to be able to walk down six flights of stairs. We developed a two-part plan whereby we notified the local fire department that a disabled resident on the sixth floor would need special assistance in case of an emergency, and two different neighbors have agreed to come check on us and assist in our evacuation should a fire or storm require it.

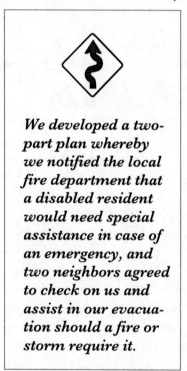

We developed a two-part plan whereby we notified the local fire department that a disabled resident would need special assistance in case of an emergency, and two neighbors agreed to check on us and assist in our evacuation should a fire or storm require it.

The therapist also had me practice getting in and out of our condo's hot tub and swimming pool—an exercise to which I did not object. Obviously both require extra caution maneuvering on slippery tile, but the benefits were certainly worth the added effort. The hot tub provided much needed relief to my almost constant arm and shoulder pain, and the pool was a great place to do my exercises while catching a few rays.

On a more mundane note, the PT also had me continue to do various exercises to maintain proper muscle tone and stamina. Since I'm a fan of watching TV, he even suggested we install a grab bar in the den so that while I watched the game I could do my deep knee bends and avoid fanny fatigue.

One of the best exercise tools he introduced to me was a specially-designed exercise bicycle. By taking the seat off of a standard issue stationary bike, I could roll up to the machine, insert my feet in a pair of tennis shoes he had cleverly bolted on to the pedals, and get plenty of good aerobic exercise from the safety of my wheelchair. It was a bit of trick to learn to get the pedals moving with just my right leg, but once I got going, my left leg was kept limber by the passive exercise, and of course I

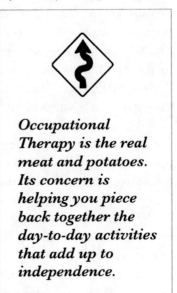

Occupational Therapy is the real meat and potatoes. Its concern is helping you piece back together the day-to-day activities that add up to independence.

could keep an eye on the television while staying fit.

A good therapist will also assure that you're outfitted with all the necessary assistive devices. I use an arm brace and a leg brace on my left side, and the therapist has several times had a specialist adjust or rebuild them to keep them in top shape. Even my wheelchair needs repair every now and then. The height of the back, the position of the arm and foot rests, the tension of the brakes, even the type of tires effect the performance and ride. I've been lucky to have a home care PT who makes sure all my gear is in top condition. He even recommended a special seat cushion that prevents sores, and suggested I get a lumbar pillow for lower back support.

As I mentioned previously, physical therapy focuses mainly on regaining your motor skills, but occupational therapy is the real meat and potatoes. It's concern is helping you piece back together the day-to-day activities that add up to independence. Getting out of bed, getting to the bathroom, taking a shower, brushing your teeth, dressing—these are the things that "occupied" me most during the early stages of my recovery.

For those readers who have not had a stroke, I'd suggest a little exercise. Try getting through a day—or even 15 minutes—using only your right hand and your right leg. Imagine you don't even have a left side—for that's what it really seems like—and try to do the simplest of things around the house. If you can resist cheating, you'll learn one overarching lesson: you have to invent whole new ways of doing things to make it work. And, everything takes a heck of a lot more time!

I was fortunate to have several good therapists—and a persistent and encouraging family—and slowly, I mean very slowly, I began to be able to do some of the necessary functions on my own.

Let's start from the beginning of a typical day. You're awake. You can almost taste that first cup of coffee. But there's the small matter of getting out of bed. Since I had one of those electric adjustable beds, the first step for me was to get the bed in a completely flat position. Plus, there was a railing on the outer edge of the mattress which helped me turn over without falling out of bed, so this had to be lowered before trying to get up. Then, as if I were some Olympic gymnast, I had to hook my strong right leg under my weak left leg, push up on the mattress with my right hand and swing my feet off the bed, all in one fluid motion. That was the farthest I could get without calling for assistance, because the next step involved standing up and moving to my wheelchair. Once help had arrived, I would first put on my slippers or shoes—trying to stand barefoot or in your socks was too slippery and dangerous. Then my wife or the home health aide would move the wheelchair into position, close alongside the bed. By the way, if you're going to try this, don't forget to lock the brakes! There's nothing worse than making your move to sit down and having the chair scoot out from under you. Once the chair was safely positioned and I was sitting on the edge of the bed, my helper would get a good grip on the ever-present gait belt. Then, with a rocking motion and a verbal count of 1-2-3, I would push up with my right hand and reach for my cane which had been positioned nearby. Once standing, and with my aide's cues, I would maneuver into position, release the cane, grab the arm of the wheelchair and carefully move into a sitting position. That's a lot to think about—and a lot of effort—just to stand up and sit down again, but transferring from the bed to my wheelchair was the gateway to the rest of the day, and I'm so grateful to my therapist for teaching me how to do it.

Once up, my first stop is typically the bathroom. A simple endeavor—something we all do a couple of times a day, right? Not so fast, Buster, if you live in a one-armed, one-legged world. First, you get your wheelchair in the right position, typically at a ninety-degree angle to the toilet. Lock those brakes, reach over with your right hand and lift your left leg off of the foot rest, pushing the metal plate out of the way. Scoot to the edge of your seat, begin the rocking motion, and, again, with the help of an aide, rise to a standing position. My son-in-law installed a grab bar at just the right height so that I could hang on to it when I was either standing or sitting. When you have a disability, modesty goes out the window. Your aide typically drops your pants and, with a firm grip on the gait belt, helps lower you to the toilet seat. Since I like to catch up on my reading while in the bathroom, we installed a cushioned toilet seat. And so that I have all of my favorite things nearby—coffee cup, newspapers, cigarettes (yes, I know)—we put a narrow shelf and magazine rack beside the toilet.

Next, I usually moved over to the sink to wash my face, brush my teeth, shave and comb my hair. Unless you're fortunate enough to have a roll-under sink, you can't approach the sink straight on because the front of the wheel chair and your legs get in the way. As long as you have a large enough bathroom to maneuver in, the best bet is to come alongside with your good arm closest to the counter. Eleanor and I realized early on that we had to relocate a number of my toiletries so that they were no longer under the counter or in the medicine cabinet. Soft soap was found to be easier to use than a bar, and a small countertop rack put my bath cloth and hand towel within easy reach. A small tray now holds my toothbrush, toothpaste, brush and comb, and we had an electrician install an extra electrical outlet on my side of the sink so that I could plug in my electric razor. It took trial and error for us to discover these few small adjustments, but every one of them can make your life a little easier.

For those of us with a disability, the days of jumping out of bed, throwing on some clothes, and dashing out the door to run some errands are over. The formerly simple act of getting dressed is now broken down into dozens of small tasks that each require careful forethought and planning. Can you still get to your dresser and closet in a wheelchair? You might have to do some re-

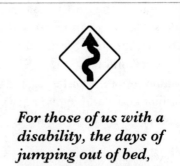

For those of us with a disability, the days of jumping out of bed, throwing on some clothes, and dashing out the door to run some errands are over. It takes a lot of planning and methodical work.

arranging. Are your old clothes hard to use now? Loose-fitting garments made of stretchable fabric are easiest to get on. All those shirts you have with buttons? Forget about it! Pullovers and v-necks with zippers are much easier. And if you wear a brace on your arm like I do, short sleeves are the way to go. Put away your belts and get some casual pants with elastic or draw-string waists. And thank God for the man who came up with Velcro to replace shoe laces! Make sure your street shoes and slippers have non-skid soles, and if you wear an AFO, you'll want to purchase shoes that are flexible enough to accommodate the extra width of the foot brace. A shoe horn is a handy thing to have around, and they even make a gadget that helps you get your socks on by spreading them at the top for you.

Although raised a Baptist, and now a part-time Presbyterian, getting dressed after a stroke makes me feel like a Catholic! Sit down to put your shirt on. Stand up to put your pants on. Sit down to put your shoes on. Stand up to transfer to the wheelchair. With all that sitting and standing, you get a pretty good workout before you've even left the bedroom!

If you plan on getting a shower, add another 30 to 45 minutes to your schedule. And make sure you have someone install plenty of sturdy grab bars in and around the shower. Don't count on using your towel racks—they're not made to support much weight.

On a day when I did the whole routine—getting up, showering, shaving and dressing—it was often two hours before I made it to the breakfast table, and by that time there was typically a therapist or a home health care worker waiting for me as I wolfed down a quick bite.

My home care occupational therapist was a real gem, teaching me many new techniques for getting around our condo. For example, just prior to the stroke we had the walls painted and wallpapered, and now every time I tried to roll from one room to another in my wheelchair I was bumping into walls, leaving black tire marks and small nicks in the paper. My OT taught me to use a spot she marked on the baseboard to gauge when it was time to start my turn so that I didn't cut the corner too tightly and bang into the wall. She continually was coming up with creative tips like this that made my life easier, and helped me be less dependent on Eleanor.

The speech therapist who worked with me at home reminded me of the Iron Lady, Margaret Thatcher. Like the former Prime Minister, she was British, and she had a way of getting me to work—hard—even when I didn't want to. The stroke left my long-term memory intact, while making it somewhat harder to remember events from the recent past, so we spent some time each session doing exercises designed to sharpen my memory. To improve my reading retention, she would have me read the day's newspaper and then answer questions about the content. There were also pronunciation problems to be overcome. For some reason I had trouble with multi-syllable words, especially those with double consonants such as "bubblegum" or "traffic light." To work on this, we created a vocabulary list of difficult words and went over them each session.

We also spent a lot of time on something I hadn't done since college, creative writing. The therapist would pose a problem, and ask me to draft a written solution. Or she would suggest a topic and I was to write a short essay expressing my opinion on the matter. At first I resented all this homework—after all, I was the former college professor—it was I who should be giving the homework. But using her personal charm and wit, not to mention that beguiling British accent, she got me to greatly improve my ability to communicate with the written word.

These in-home therapists were true professionals, and several of them became friends. One day when I was doing exercises with my occupational therapist, I confided in her that when I had my stroke, I really didn't understand what had happened to me. I had been given CAT scans and MRIs, and told it was a stroke, but I understood very little about what caused it and what the aftermath would entail. I was somewhat relieved but also horrified when she said that, of the past 100 or so patients she had worked with, almost none of them had a very clear sense of what a stroke is, nor had they been clearly pre-pared for the months and years of hard work that lay ahead of them on the road to recovery. This conversation made me all the more sure that a book for patients and their families which explained stroke in plain language was a necessity.

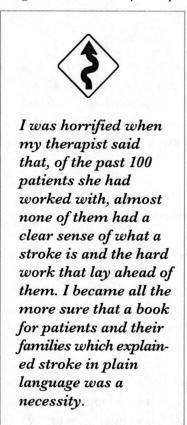

I was horrified when my therapist said that, of the past 100 patients she had worked with, almost none of them had a clear sense of what a stroke is and the hard work that lay ahead of them. I became all the more sure that a book for patients and their families which explained stroke in plain language was a necessity.

Chapter 19
COPING WITH PAIN

Amidst all the coming and going of the various therapists and health care workers, there was one regular but uninvited guest—pain. Even though I had largely lost the use of my left arm, I hadn't lost the ability to feel pain. Day in and day out—and especially at night—I experienced intense discomfort in my arm and shoulder.

After trying the usual Tylenol™ and Advil™ to no avail, I knew something else had to be done, so to my already burgeoning roster of Doctors was added a variety of pain specialists. First, I went to an anesthesiologist who was reported to have had success in some patients with a series of Lidocaine™ shots. My hopes for relief were dashed when he decided to discontinue the treatment after only two injections. When I complained that he had stopped prematurely, he said, "If it were going to work, it would have worked by now. You may just have to live with it." Not what I wanted to hear. Hope found—hope lost.

Next, I had an x-ray which revealed no abnormalities. "It's the stroke," replied the technician. "Get used to it." I flashed back to one of the slogans of the Clinton/Bush race—"It's the economy, stupid."

The first treatment that actually seemed to work was a time-release patch. After several weeks, the pain had noticeably lessened, yet my wife reported that I was periodically having unusual thoughts and talking in a confused manner. Hope found—hope lost, once again.

We did some research regarding advanced pain medication, but when I asked my doctor to prescribe several of the newer pills, he said that, while effective, they were also known to be addictive. My pain-free search continued.

This time I turned to alternative medicine—acupuncture. On my initial visit, the acupuncturist informed me that he thought he could help. Hope, again. After several appointments, he reviewed my MRI, and on the following visit told me that the stroke had done so much damage to my brain that he did not feel continued treatment would be helpful. Hope lost.

Through all of this, I was sporadically praying for relief, though I wasn't sure it was right to ask God for a miracle since we hadn't been in touch all that much lately. My son arranged a meeting with a college friend who was now a local pastor. The session in his office was a little unnerving, but he assured me I had no need to feel hesitant about asking God for a miracle. After a brief time of prayer together, I left, notably relieved, and I think I even experienced less pain for a couple of days until it returned.

The doctors told me there were only two more options. One was a treatment that hadn't been used for years but was making a comeback. You went into the hospital and they injected your entire body with Novocain™, the numbing medication often used by dentists. The other option was to go to the famed Mayo Pain Clinic and let them put a shunt in your brain which administered medication into your neural system at regular intervals. The thought of having them shave my head and open up my brain was just too much, and I began to think that the first doctor had been right. I was just going to have to learn to live with it.

As luck would have it, after going from pillar to post seeing specialists all over town, the relief I was seeking was finally found right under my nose. During a regularly-scheduled follow-up visit with my neurologist, he prescribed two Elavil™ tablets each night at bedtime and moist heat applied to the arm and shoulder twice daily. Within a week the pain began subsiding.

Finally, this unwelcome guest had taken its leave. Yet it wasn't long before another more troublesome visitor took its place—depression.

STROKE

Chapter 20
DEALING WITH DEPRESSION

*T*he *Merck Manual of Medical Information* defines depression as "a feeling of intense sadness that is out of proportion to the event that caused it," and one that "persists beyond an appropriate length of time."[1] Although before the stroke I had had my share of disappointments and sorrows, I wouldn't have thought of myself as depressed. As time passed, I began to be more aware of what the stroke had cost me in terms of freedom, mobility and overall quality of life. I now spent most of my time either in bed or in the

Some of the common effects of stroke include sleeplessness, exhaustion, irritability, emotional outbursts, inconsolable sadness, an unwillingness to communicate, despair, and suicidal thoughts. Believe me, I've experienced them all.

wheelchair, and the resultant lethargy gave me too much time to think about my losses.

I tried talking to my wife and my children about it, but I felt like I was already such a drain on them that I didn't want to bring them down emotionally, too. I talked with some of my former students who had remained good friends. I talked to my pastor and to God. But the feelings of despondency continued.

When I mentioned it to one of my therapists, she said I had every right to be depressed. She explained that in addition to the loss of some physical function, it was also very typical for stroke victims to feel depressed because of chemical changes in their brains. For example, she said that if the stroke occurred in the area of the brain that controls emotions, some patients experience periods of involuntary and uncontrollable crying. Alternately, some are seized with fits of laughter or outbursts of bad temper. I recalled that one of my fellow patients at the rehab hospital would often say only one word, "shit." An entire conversation might consist of her simply repeating over and over—"Shit, shit, shit." (Although I didn't say it, I often felt it.) I've read that other common effects of stroke include sleeplessness, exhaustion, irritability, emotional outbursts, inconsolable sadness, an unwillingness to communicate, despair and suicidal thoughts. Believe me, I've experienced them all.

My primary care physician and neurologist referred me to a local psychiatrist who, with very little conversation as to my feelings and the possible causes of my depression, began prescribing one antidepressant after another. During subsequent visits he would either adjust my dosage or switch me to another pill like some kind of guinea pig. The most consistent reaction I had as a result of all of those different medications was nausea.

I had always heard that the best results when dealing with emotional problems were achieved by a combination of medication and counseling, but remembering the disappointing results with my counselor at the rehab hospital and my distaste for group therapy, I didn't know where to turn. Finally my psychiatrist suggested that I meet with a counselor on his staff, and with some reluctance I went in for a session of "talking therapy." To my surprise, and elation, we hit it off. There was just something about his manner that made me feel free to talk, and even when we didn't discuss my condition per se, I always left feeling a little better.

To date I've still found no magic pill, and I can't say that there have been any big psychological breakthroughs. But the combination of medication and talk does seem to help me keep my head above water—most of the time. Even to this day I struggle with periodic bouts of despair. Suicide is such an ugly thought, but it does hold the appeal of bringing a quick end to all of your problems. I know my wife is correct when she says it would be a very selfish act, and I've never planned a serious attempt. I've got to confess, however, that in some ways the depression that often comes with a stroke can be more debilitating than the brain attack, itself.

---

[1] *The Merck Manual of Medical Information: Home Edition;* p.403; M. Beers, A. Fletcher, T. Jones, R. Porter, M. Berkwits; Paw Prints 2008

STROKE

Chapter 21
CLOSING THE GAP BETWEEN
THEORY & EXPERIENCE

E ven though I had known and worked with handicapped people all of my professional life, I still was not prepared for what it actually felt like to have a disability. Often I've wished I could restart my career in special education and use all of the insights I've gained since my stroke.

Likewise, I suspect that most people involved in helping the disabled find it nearly impossible to really know what they're going through. For example, many medical personnel who initially began their careers out of a heartfelt desire to help people, may find themselves, as they

The most difficult part of having a stroke is not the struggle to learn to walk again, nor to think and speak more clearly, nor to regain lost skills. The most difficult part of having a stroke is accepting what it has done to your mind and body.

137

pursue technical expertise and professional growth, distracted from their original motivation. As they go deeper into the arcanum of their field, many find themselves better equipped to talk with other physicians than with their patients. Financial and scheduling pressures at their practices can inadvertently chip away at their bedside manner until an appointment with a patient is reduced to a brief flurry of technobabble followed by a script. "Slam. Bam. Take your pills, Ma'am."

Family members who either choose to or find themselves serving a loved one as their primary caregiver rightly need to learn all they can about the patient's condition and the therapies that may help them improve. That alone can consume your energies 24 hours a day, 7 days a week. But one mustn't let the patient's physical needs distract you from their very real, but perhaps hidden, emotional needs.

For many who have suffered a disability as the result of a traumatic accident or illness, it takes months, even years, for the full impact of the damage done to sink in. And when it does, it leaves an indelible imprint upon your emotions. The most difficult part of having a stroke is not the struggle to learn to walk again, nor to think and speak more clearly, nor to regain lost skills. The most difficult part of having a stroke is accepting what it has done to your mind and body.

I know that, to some extent, my left neglect kept me from really coming to terms with my disabilities. Somehow, the part of my brain that was damaged kept me from recognizing that I had lost most of the use of my left arm and leg. When, over the course of time, I realized I was seriously handicapped—like so many children I had worked with—the subsequent turmoil was powerful. I felt sick, anxious, dejected, depressed and cheated. Like so many before me, I asked, "Why me, God, why me? What have I done to deserve this? Why are you punishing me?" You ponder, "How can I become normal again? What will my future be? Do I even have a future? Who will help me through this?"

I know now that my sense of despair and hopelessness is shared by millions of people around the world—people struck out of the blue by some debilitating disease. Many people turn to the well-known "Serenity Prayer" for solace. "God grant me the serenity to accept the things I cannot change, courage to change the things I can, and wisdom to know the difference." I feel like I've done fairly well in the courage department—my extensive physical, occupational, speech and psychological therapy

To the hundreds of thousands of others whose lives have been turned upside down by stroke, I can only say that the road ahead is long, winding, and often damned hard.

have taken a great deal of courage, time and hard work. But I cannot find the wisdom to know the difference between what I can and cannot change. And I cannot accept what the stroke has done to me, no matter how hard I try.

I appreciate the investment my many doctors and therapists have made in me. Likewise, the love and encouragement from many friends and family members—especially my son and daughter and their families—have meant a lot. Words cannot express the deep debt of gratitude I owe my wife, Eleanor, for sacrificing her life for mine.

To the hundreds of thousands of others whose lives have been turned upside down by stroke or another devastating disease, I can only say that the road ahead is long, winding, and often damned hard. May you be as blessed as I to have people willing to walk with you, for the road to recovery—like the road of love—goes on forever.

EPILOGUE

K nowing how to conclude a book like this is just as hard as starting it. I am by no means finished with my recovery, and have no pat answers or victory speeches to offer. I can report that, nearly six years after my stroke, a round of **MRIs** and **EEGs** confirmed that there had been no subsequent stroke activity—a relief to us all.

One other development has been that we received the shocking news not too long ago that my great granddaughter, Natalie, had suffered a stroke—at age 13 months! Imagine our dismay! While playing on her indoor swing set, Natalie fell and hit her head. Based on initial symptoms, it seemed like just another childhood accident. But when her mother, Lisa (my daughter's daughter), noticed that she was not using her left arm or leg, she feared the worst and rushed her to the hospital.

A CT scan confirmed that the fall had sheared an artery in an area near the base of Natalie's brain called the basal ganglia. Further tests revealed that she had paralysis from the left side of her mouth all the way down to her toes. Having been to visit me numerous times since my stroke, I'm sure Lisa and her husband imagined that now their tiny daughter, too, would lead a life plagued with disabilities.

Thankfully, after only a few days in the hospital, Natalie's facial paralysis disappeared, and she showed signs of slight movement in her left hand. With that encouragement, the doctors put her on a four-day-a-week schedule of physical therapy, just like her "Great Big D." Less than a month after the stroke, Natalie took her first steps—again. She had just learned to walk immediately prior to the accident, and thankfully what started as a slow wobble once again became the excited patter of little feet heading into a bright future.

Surprisingly, Natalie's stroke is not that rare. Recent reports show that the incidence of stroke in children under 14 is about 3 per 100,000, and that 28% of all strokes occur in people under the age of 65. The prospects for youngsters who suffer an injury in the basal ganglia like Natalie are good. One study by Doctors Dharker, Mittal and Bhargava found that of 23 children under the age of six-and-a-half years who suffered paralysis on one side of their bodies, all but one recovered completely within four months.[1]

Thankfully, Natalie is living a healthy life now, but the incident serves as a dramatic reminder that all of us who have loved ones who have suffered a stroke, or who have experienced one ourselves, need to constantly be learning all we can about stroke prevention, rehabilitation and recovery. To that end, we hope this book has been of some help to you and your loved ones.

---

[1] "Journal of Neurology, Neurosurgery and Psychology," volume 73(1), July 2002.

POSTSCRIPT

After nine long years of struggling with stroke, Dr. Prillaman passed away—not from stroke, but from a cancerous brain tumor. His love and humor are deeply missed, but he will forever be appreciated by his wife, children, grandchildren, friends and loved ones. His was, indeed, a life well lived.

STROKE

UNDERSTANDING STROKE: AN *EXPERIENTIAL* GUIDE TO MEDICAL TERMINOLOGY

Following are some of the strange, new words you will undoubtedly encounter as you and your loved ones cope with stroke. They are listed here in the order you might hear them come up. This section is followed by an alphabetical listing.

- **Stroke**

  A Stroke occurs when blood flow to the brain is interrupted. It could be caused by an Artery getting blocked (an Ischemic Stroke) or by a blood vessel bursting (a Hemorrhagic Stroke). Blood provides the oxygen and nutrients the brain needs to function, and when blood flow is interrupted the brain cells in the immediate area begin to die. Depending on the area and extent of the brain damage, certain abilities such as speech, movement and clear thinking can be lost.

Types of Stroke

- **Ischemic Stroke**

  About 80% of strokes are caused by the blockage of an Artery or other vessel that carries blood to the brain. If a Blood Clot (or Thrombus) forms where the vessel is clogged, it's call a Thrombotic Stroke. If a blood clot forms somewhere else in the body and then travels (an Embolus or Embolism) to the clogged area, it's called an Embolic Stroke.

- **Hemorrhagic Stroke**

  About 20% of strokes are caused by bleeding into the brain. A blood vessel may have grown weak and enlarged like a balloon to the point of bursting (an Aneurysm), or there may have been a cluster of abnormally formed blood vessels (an AVM, or Arteriovenous Malformation) that got tangled up and caused bleeding into the brain. In either case, the leaking blood puts pressure on the brain, causing damage.

- **Transient Ischemic Attack (TIA)**

  A third type of stroke is called a Transient Ischemic Attack, or TIA. These occur when a blood clot causes a temporary blockage, and then dissolves or passes through. TIAs, often called "mini-strokes," seldom cause lasting damage. However, they should be taken seriously, and are sometimes called "warning strokes."

Locations of Strokes

As the location of a stroke determines what part of the brain may be damaged—and what types of disabilities might be experienced—understanding the anatomy of the brain can help.

Your brain has three main sections: the Cerebrum, the Cerebellum and the Brain Stem.

- **Cerebrum**

  The Cerebrum is the largest and most advanced part of the brain. It is divided into two Hemispheres, or halves—Left and Right. Because of how we're wired, the Left Hemisphere controls the right side of the body, and the Right Hemisphere controls the left side of the body. The Cerebrum also has four sections called the Cerebral Lobes. Going front to back, they're called the Frontal Lobe, the Parietal Lobes, the Temporal Lobes and the Occipital Lobe.

  - **Frontal Lobe**

    The Frontal Lobe allows us to plan, organize, and solve problems. A portion of it, the Prefrontal Cortex, controls personality, emotions and behavior. The back of the Frontal Lobe produces movement.

  - **Parietal Lobes**

    The Left and Right Parietal Lobes are sections of the brain behind the Frontal Lobe that control sensation, including touch.

- Plus, the **Right Parietal Lobe** effects what's called "visuo-spatial perception"—the ability for us to find our way around.

- The **Left Parietal Lobe** helps us understand language—both spoken and written.

o **Temporal Lobes**
The Left and Right Temporal Lobes, down near your ears, help us distinguish smells and sounds.

- Plus, the **Right Temporal Lobe** is involved in visual memory (things you've seen) and short term memory.

- The **Left Temporal Lobe** is involved in verbal memory (things you've heard, including words and names of people, places and things).

o **Occipital Lobe**
The Occipital Lobe handles visual perception, and helps us recognize shapes and colors.

- **Cerebellum**

  The Cerebellum is located at the back of the brain and is the second largest section. It effects your reflexes, balance and certain aspects of your coordination.

- **Brain Stem**

  The Brain Stem is at the bottom of the brain where it connects to the spinal cord. It handles many of the "automatic" functions of your body such as breathing, your heartbeat, digestion and being awake.

  The "Stroke Resources" section that follows features links to several online illustrations of brain anatomy. See page 185 and following.

Testing for Stroke

If a person is exhibiting signs of Stroke (sudden weakness, confusion, trouble speaking or seeing), get them to the hospital right away. Time is of the essence. Once in the Emergency Room, the staff may administer any number of tests.

- **MRI—Magnetic Resonance Imaging**

  An MRI uses a large magnetic field to produce an image of the brain that allows doctors to determine the location and extent of the injury.

- **EEG—Electroencephalogram**

  An EEG reads the brain waves through small discs placed on the head.

- **Ultrasound**
  Ultrasound measures the flow of blood in arteries. The three main kinds are called B-mode Imaging, Doppler Testing and Duplex Scanning.

- **MRA—Magnetic Resonance Angiography**
  Doctors can inject a small amount of die into a blood vessel and then X-Ray the area to observe how the blood is flowing.

Effects of Stroke

Depending on which part of your brain suffers a stroke, you may experience some of the following problems.

Problems with Movement

- **Paralysis**
  Loss of movement of certain muscles or limbs.

- **Hemiplegia**
  Paralysis on only one side of the body.

- **Paresis**
  Not complete Paralysis, but weakness of muscles.

- **Hemiparesis**
  Weakness on one side of the body.

- **Apraxia**
  The inability to put together the right combination of muscle movements.

- **Ataxia**
  A lack of coordination, unsteadiness.

- **Spasticity**
  Abnormal contraction of muscles.

- **Spastic Paralysis**
  Paralysis with increased contraction of muscles.

- **Dysarthria**
  Although it seems like a Speech problem, Dysarthria is actually a muscle problem in the tongue, mouth, voice box or jaw that makes it hard to speak clearly.

- **Dysphagia**
  Difficulty or inability to swallow.

Problems with Communicating

- **Dysphasia**
  Trouble understanding or creating words.

- **Aphasia**
  The loss of the power of expression or comprehension of speech or writing. The two main types are named after the doctors who discovered the specific areas of the brain which, when damaged by stroke, cause the disorder.

- **Broca's Aphasia**
  People with Broca's Aphasia may be able to understand what words mean, but have trouble

physically forming them.

- **Wernicke's Aphasia**
  People with Wernicke's Aphasia may be able to make sounds, even words, but have trouble putting them in the right order.

- **Agraphia**
  The inability to write.

- **Alexia**
  The inability to read.

Problems with Perception

- **Anosognosia**
  The lack of awareness or denial that anything is wrong with the stroke-affected side of the body.

- **Neglect**
  The lack of awareness of one side of your body.

- **Hemianopia**
  The loss of half the field of vision in each eye.

- **Dementia**
  A decrease or loss of mental ability.

- **Agnosia**
  Difficulty recognizing objects or persons, or understanding the meaning of sensory stimuli such as touch, sounds and smells.

Treatment for Stroke

Getting the necessary treatment for stroke involves dealing with physicians, nurses, specialists, therapists, and a host of people and things that have funny initials. Here's a quick overview.

Doctors and Nurses

- **Triage Nurse**

  The first person you'll likely see when you enter the Emergency Room. Determines the severity of each patient's symptoms and the priority in which they will be helped.

- **Emergency Room Physician**

  The doctor who provides initial testing and care and who may refer you for admission into the main Hospital.

- **Physician**

  A medical doctor, either a general practitioner (GP) or a specialist.

- **Neurologist**

  A physician who specializes in the function of the brain, nervous system, muscles and spinal cord.

- **Nurse**

  A broad term for a group of healthcare professionals who, in collaboration with physicians and others, are responsible to assess, plan, implement and evaluate your medical care.

- **Charge Nurse**
  A registered nurse (RN) who oversees all nursing and assistive staff.

- **Nurse Practitioner**
  An RN who has either a Masters or Doctoral degree and can prescribe medicines.

- **Registered Nurse (RN)**
  A nurse who has graduated from a 4-year College or Nursing School.

- **Licensed Practical Nurse (LPN)**
  A nurse with a 1- or 2-year degree from a community college or technical school.

- **Licensed Vocational Nurse (LVN)**
  See Licensed Practical Nurse, above.

- **Certified Nursing Assistant (CNA or CVA)**
  An unlicensed assistive staff person.

Specialists and Therapists

- **Neurologist**
  A brain specialist.

- **Cardiologist**
  A heart doctor.

- **Urologist**
  A bladder and urinary tract doctor.

- **Nephrologists**
A kidney doctor.

- **Respiratory Therapist**
A breathing specialist.

- **Physical Therapist (PT)**
Works with patients to help them with movement, especially walking.

- **Occupational Therapist (OT)**
Helps restore one's ability to do ADLs—the Activities of Daily Living—with concentration on upper body skills.

- **Speech Pathologist**
Helps you with language and communication skills.

- **Recreational Therapist**
Provides physical and emotional therapy through play.

- **Psychologist**
Can help a patient deal with the changes in their life through counseling.

- **Psychiatrist**
A medical doctor who can prescribe medication to help patients who are struggling emotionally.

- **Dietician**
Plans your food and nutrition.

- **Case Manager**
  A worker at a Hospital who coordinates a patient's therapies.

Levels of Care in Hospitals

- **Stroke Unit**
  A dedicated area of a hospital staffed by doctors and nurses who specialize in stroke treatment.

- **Intensive Care (Critical Care)**
  The highest level of treatment and monitoring.

- **Progressive Care**
  Once a patient has begun to improve, they may be "stepped down" to progressive care.

Types of Facilities

- **Emergency Room**
  Get there immediately if you've experienced stroke symptoms.

- **Hospital**
  A local or regional facility that provides staff and equipment for medical, surgical and nursing treatment.

- **Rehabilitation Hospital**
  After a stroke patient has been diagnosed, treated and stabilized in a hospital, they may be moved to a Rehab Hospital in order to regain mobility, strength, and as many of their pre-stroke abilities

as they can.

- **Inpatient Care**
  When a patient stays overnight at a Hospital.

- **Outpatient Care**
  When a patient comes to a Hospital for only a few hours each day to get treatment.

- **Nursing Home (Rest Home, Skilled Nursing Unit)**
  Once a patient has benefited all they can from therapy and rehabilitation, they may live in a nursing home where they can get around-the-clock care.

Acronyms and Abbreviations

- **ADLs (Activities of Daily Living)**
  Bathing, grooming, dressing, cooking, etc.

- **AFO (Ankle-Foot Orthotic)**
  A device that supports or corrects the function of a stroke-affected foot.

- **Cath (Catheter)**
  A tube that can be inserted to either drain or administer fluids.

- **CNA**
  A Certified Nursing Assistant.

- **CT Scan (or Cat Scan)**
  A Computed Tomography Scan.

- **CVA (Cerebrovascular Accident)**
  A Stroke.

- **DNR (Do Not Resuscitate)**
  A legal document, sometimes called a Living Will, stating that a patient does not want to be resuscitated if they suffer a cardiac or respiratory arrest.

- **ECG (Electrocardiogram)**
  A non-invasive way to check a person's heart.

- **EEG (Electroencephalogram)**
  A non-invasive way to check a person's brain.

- **ICU (Intensive Care Unit) or CCU (Critical Care Unit)**
  A section of a Hospital especially equipped with life support and care for the critically ill.

- **LPN (Licensed Practical Nurse)**
  A mid-level nurse.

- **LVN (Licensed Vocational Nurse)**
  Same as LPN.

- **MRA (Magnetic Resonance Angiography)**
  A way to see blood vessels, especially arteries in the brain.

- **MRI (Magnetic Resonance Imaging)**
A non-invasive test that produces images using large magnets.

- **OT (Occupational Therapy)**
Concerned with restoring "activities of daily living."

- **PT (Physical Therapy)**
Concerned with restoring movement, especially walking.

- **RN (Registered Nurse)**
A senior nurse.

- **TIA (Transient Ischemic Attack)**
A short-lasting "mini-stroke."

Other Key Terms

- **Anoxia**
When blood flow is cut off and almost no oxygen gets to a cell, potentially causing cell death.

- **Artery**
A blood vessel that carries blood away from the heart to the rest of the body.

- **Aspirate**
To breathe food or other matter into the lungs.

- **Blood Clot**
When blood has changed from its normal liquid

state to a solid state. It's also called a Thrombus.

- **Carotid Arteries**
Two Arteries, running along the left and right sides of your neck, that supply the head and neck with blood.

- **Cerebrovascular**
Concerning the blood vessels that feed the brain.

- **Cue**
To give someone verbal instruction to remind them what to do.

- **Edema**
A swelling. Sometimes spelled Oedema.

- **Embolism**
When a blood vessel is blocked by a blood clot that has traveled through the bloodstream.

- **Gait Belt**
A belt used by nurses and therapists to help someone stand and walk.

- **Hematoma**
When collected blood causes swelling which can put pressure on and damage the brain. Sometimes spelled Haematoma.

- **Hemorrhage**
Bleeding. Sometimes spelled Haemorrhage.

- **Hypoxia**
  When a cell receives lowered levels of oxygen.

- **Infarct**
  An area of brain tissue that has died due to lack of oxygen. Sometimes called an Infarction.

- **Intubate**
  To insert tubes.

- **Ischemia**
  A severe reduction or loss of blood flow. Sometimes spelled Ischaemia.

- **Ischemic Cascade**
  A series of reactions in the brain in which one reduction in blood flow triggers the next.

- **Ischemic Penumbra**
  An area of still-living cells near an Ischemia.

- **Motor Function**
  The ability to move, especially to walk.

- **Occlude**
  To close up.

- **Stenosis**
  The narrowing of an artery.

- **Subarachnoid Hemorrhage**
  Bleeding between the brain and the thin tissues that cover the brain.

- **Syncope**
  Partial or complete loss of consciousness.

- **Thromboembolus**
  A clot which has traveled to a blocked artery or vein.

- **Thrombosis**
  The formation of a blood clot, sometimes called a Thrombus.

- **Tone**
  Referring to the contraction of muscles.

- **Vascular**
  Our system of blood vessels, including Arteries, Veins and Capillaries.

- **Vein**
  A blood vessel that carries blood back to the heart.

- **Vertebral Arteries**
  Two Arteries that come up from the spinal column to the brain.

UNDERSTANDING STROKE: AN *ALPHABETICAL* GUIDE TO MEDICAL TERMINOLOGY

ADLs (Activities of Daily Living)
Bathing, grooming, dressing, cooking, etc.

AFO (Ankle-Foot Orthotic)
A device that supports or corrects the function of a stroke-affected foot.

Agnosia
Difficulty recognizing objects or persons, or understanding the meaning of sensory stimuli such as touch, sounds and smells.

Agraphia
The inability to write.

Alexia
The inability to read.

Aneurysm
When a blood vessel grows weak and enlarges like a balloon to the point of bursting.

Anosognosia
The lack of awareness or denial that anything is wrong with the stroke-affected side of the body.

Anoxia
When blood flow is cut off and almost no oxygen gets to a cell, potentially causing cell death.

Aphasia
The loss of the power of expression or comprehension of speech or writing.

Apraxia
Unable to put together the right combination of muscle movements.

Arteriovenous Malformation
See AVM.

Artery
A blood vessel that carries blood away from the heart to the rest of the body.

Aspirate
To breathe food or other matter into the lungs.

Ataxia
A lack of coordination, unsteadiness.

AVM (Arteriovenous Malformation)
A cluster of abnormally formed blood vessels that got tangled up and caused bleeding into the brain.

Blood Clot
When blood has changed from its normal liquid state to a solid state. It's also called a Thrombus.

Brain Stem
The Brain Stem is at the bottom of the brain where it connects to the spinal cord. It handles many of the "automatic" functions of your body such as breathing, your heartbeat, digestion and being awake.

Broca's Aphasia
People with Broca's Aphasia may be able to understand what words mean, but have trouble physically forming them.

Cardiologist
A heart Doctor.

Carotid Arteries
Two Arteries, running along the left and right sides of your neck, that supply the head and neck with blood.

Case Manager
A worker at a Hospital that coordinates a patient's therapies.

Cat Scan
See CT Scan.

Cath (Catheter)
A tube that can be inserted to either drain or administer fluids.

CCU (Critical Care Unit)

A section of a Hospital especially equipped with life support and care for the critically ill. Sometimes called ICU.

Cerebellum

The Cerebellum is located at the back of the brain and is the second largest section. It effects your reflexes, balance and certain aspects of your coordination.

Cerebral Lobes

The four sections of the Cerebrum.

Cerebrovascular

Concerning the blood vessels that feed the brain.

Cerebrum

The Cerebrum is the largest and most advanced part of the brain. It is divided into two hemispheres, or halves— Left and Right. Because of how we're wired, the Left Hemisphere controls the right side of the body, and the Right Hemisphere controls the left side of the body. The Cerebrum also has four sections called the Cerebral Lobes. Going front to back, they're called the Frontal Lobe, the Parietal Lobes, the Temporal Lobes and the Occipital Lobe.

Certified Nursing Assistant (CNA or CVA)

An unlicensed assistive staff person.

Charge Nurse

A registered nurse (RN) who oversees all nursing and assistive staff.

CNA
A certified nursing assistant.

Critical Care Unit
See CCU.

CT Scan (or Cat Scan)
A computed tomography scan.

Cue
To give someone verbal instruction to remind them what to do.

CVA (Cerebrovascular Accident)
A stroke.

Dementia
A decrease or loss of mental ability.

Dietician
A person at a hospital or rehab facility who plans your food and nutrition.

DNR (Do Not Resuscitate)
A legal document, sometimes called a living will, stating that a patient does not want to be resuscitated if they suffer a cardiac or respiratory arrest.

Dysarthria
Although it seems like a speech problem, dysarthria is actually a muscle problem in the tongue, mouth, voice-box or jaw that makes it hard to speak clearly.

Dysphagia
Difficulty or inability to swallow.

Dysphasia
Trouble understanding or creating words.

ECG (Electrocardiogram)
A non-invasive way to check a person's heart.

Edema
A swelling. Sometimes spelled Oedema.

EEG (Electroencephalogram)
An EEG reads the brain waves through small discs placed on the head.

Electrocardiogram
See ECG.

Electroencephalogram
See EEG.

Embolic Stroke
When a Blood Clot forms somewhere else in the body and then travels (an Embolus or Embolism) to a clogged blood vessel, depleting the brain of blood.

Embolism
When a blood vessel is blocked by a Blood Clot that has traveled through the bloodstream.

Emergency Room
Get there immediately if you've experienced stroke symptoms.

Emergency Room Physician
The doctor who provides initial testing and care and who may refer you for admission into the main Hospital.

Frontal Lobe
The first part of the Cerebrum, which allows us to plan, organize and solve problems. A portion of it, the Prefrontal Cortex, controls personality, emotions and behavior. The back of the Frontal Lobe produces movement.

Gait Belt
A belt used by nurses and therapists to help someone stand and walk.

Hematoma
When collected blood causes swelling which can put pressure on and damage the brain. Sometimes spelled Haematoma.

Hemi-
Half.

Hemianopia
The loss of half the field of vision in each eye.

Hemiparesis
Weakness on one side of the body.

Hemiplegia
Paralysis on only one side of the body.

Hemorrhage
Bleeding. Sometimes spelled Haemorrhage.

Hemorrhagic Stroke
About 20% of strokes are caused by bleeding into the brain. A blood vessel may have grown weak and enlarged like a balloon to the point of bursting (an Aneurysm), or there may have been a cluster of abnormally formed blood vessels (an AVM, or Arteriovenous Malformation) that got tangled up and caused bleeding into the brain. In either case, the leaking blood puts pressure on the brain, causing damage.

Home Health Care
Therapies delivered at home by a healthcare professional.

Hospital
A local or regional facility that provides staff and equipment for medical, surgical and nursing treatment.

Hypoxia
When a cell receives lowered levels of oxygen.

ICU (Intensive Care Unit)
A section of a Hospital especially equipped with life support and care for the critically ill. Sometimes called CCU.

Infarct
An area of brain tissue that has died due to lack of oxygen.

Sometimes called an Infarction.

Inpatient Care
When a patient stays overnight at a Hospital.

Intensive Care (ICU)
The highest level of treatment and monitoring. Sometimes called Critical Care.

Intubate
To insert tubes.

Ischemia
A severe reduction or loss of blood flow. Sometimes spelled Ischaemia.

Ischemic Cascade
A series of reactions in the brain in which one reduction in blood flow triggers the next.

Ischemic Penumbra
An area of still-living cells near an Ischemia.

Ischemic Stroke
About 80% of strokes are caused by the blockage of an Artery or other vessel that carries blood to the brain. If a Blood Clot (or Thrombus) forms where the vessel is clogged, it's call a Thrombotic Stroke. If a blood clot forms somewhere else in the body and then travels (an Embolus or Embolism) to the clogged area, it's called an Embolic Stroke.

Left Hemisphere
The left half of the brain.

Left Parietal Lobe
Helps us understand language—both spoken and written.

Left Temporal Lobe
Involved in verbal memory (things you've heard, including words and names of people, places and things).

Licensed Practical (LPN)
A nurse with a 1- or 2-year degree from a community college or technical school.

Licensed Vocational Nurse (LVN)
Same as Licensed Practical Nurse, above.

Living Will
A legal document, sometimes called a DNR, stating that a patient does not want to be resuscitated if they suffer a cardiac or respiratory arrest.

LPN
See Licensed Practical Nurse.

LVN
See Licensed Vocational Nurse.

Motor Function
The ability to move, especially to walk.

MRA – Magnetic Resonance Angiography
Doctors can inject a small amount of dye into a blood

vessel and then X-Ray the area to observe how the blood is flowing.

MRI - Magnetic Resonance Imaging
An MRI uses a large magnetic field to produce an image of the brain that allows doctors to determine the location and extent of the injury.

Neglect
The lack of awareness of one side of your body.

Nephrologist
A kidney doctor.

Neurologist
A physician who specializes in the function of the brain, nervous system, muscles and spinal cord.

Nurse
A healthcare professional who, in collaboration with physicians and others, is responsible to assess, plan, implement and evaluate your medical care.

Nurse Practitioner
An RN who has either a Masters or Doctoral degree and can prescribe medicines.

Nursing Home (Rest Home, Skilled Nursing Unit)
Once a patient has benefited all they can from therapy and Rehabilitation, they may live in a nursing home where they can get around-the-clock care.

Occipital Lobe
The Occipital Lobe handles visual perception, and helps us recognize shapes and colors.

Occlude
To close up.

Occupational Therapist (OT)
Helps restore your ability to do ADLs—the Activities of Daily Living.

Oedema
A swelling. Sometimes spelled Edema.

OT
See Occupational Therapist.

Outpatient Care
When a patient comes to a Facility for only a few hours each day to get treatment.

Paralysis
Loss of movement of certain muscles or limbs.

Paresis
Not complete Paralysis, but weakness of muscles.

Parietal Lobes
The Left and Right Parietal Lobes are sections of the brain behind the Frontal Lobe that control sensation, including touch.

Physical Therapist (PT)
Works with patients to help restore movement, especially walking.

Physician
A full-on medical doctor, either a General Practitioner (GP) or a specialist.

Prefrontal Cortex
The area of the brain that controls personality, emotions and behavior.

Progressive Care
Once a patient has begun to improve, they may be "stepped down" from Intensive Care to Progressive Care.

Psychiatrist
A medical doctor who can prescribe medication to help patients with emotional problems.

Psychologist
Can help a patient deal with the changes in their life through counseling.

PT
(see Physical Therapist)

Recreational Therapist
Provides physical and emotional therapy through play.

Registered Nurse (RN)
A nurse who has graduated from a 4-year College or Nursing School.

Rehab Facility
See Rehabilitation Hospital.

Rehabilitation
The process of improving a stroke patient's mental and motor function.

Rehabilitation Hospital
After a stroke patient has been diagnosed, treated and stabilized in a hospital, they may be moved to a Rehab Hospital in order to regain mobility, strength, and as many of their pre-stroke abilities as they can.

Respiratory Therapist
A breathing specialist.

Right Hemisphere
The right half of the brain.

Right Parietal Lobe
Effects what's called "visuo-spatial perception"—the ability for us to find our way around.

Right Temporal Lobe
Involved in visual memory (things you've seen) and short term memory.

RN
See Registered Nurse.

Spastic Paralysis
Paralysis with increased contraction of muscles.

Spasticity
Abnormal contraction of muscles.

Speech Pathologist
Helps you with language and communication skills.

Stenosis
The narrowing of an Artery.

Stroke
A stroke occurs when blood flow to the brain is interrupted. It could be caused by an Artery getting blocked (an Ischemic Stroke) or by a blood vessel bursting (a Hemorrhagic Stroke). Blood provides the oxygen and nutrients the brain needs to function, and when blood flow is interrupted the brain cells in the immediate area begin to die. Depending on the area and extent of the brain damage, certain abilities such as speech, movement and clear thinking can be lost.

Stroke Unit
A dedicated area of a hospital staffed by physicians and s who specialize in stroke treatment.

Subarachnoid Hemorrhage
Bleeding between the brain and the thin tissues that cover the brain.

Syncope
Partial or complete loss of consciousness.

Temporal Lobes
The Left and Right Temporal Lobes, down near your

ears, help us distinguish smells and sounds.

Therapists
Hospital, Rehab Facility and Home Health Care staff who work with you on recovering lost function.

Therapy
Help administered by various specialists to aid a patient in regaining lost function.

Thromboembolus
A Blood Clot which has traveled to a blocked an Artery or vein.

Thrombosis
The formation of a Blood Clot, sometimes called a Thrombus.

Thrombotic Stroke
When a Blood Clot (or Thrombus) forms where a blood vessel is clogged, depleting the brain of blood.

Thrombus
A Blood Clot.

TIA
See Transient Ischemic Attack.

Tone
Referring to the contraction of muscles.

Transient Ischemic Attack (TIA)
A third type of stroke is called a Transient Ischemic

Attack, or TIA. These occur when a Blood Clot causes a temporary blockage, and then dissolves or passes through. TIAs, often called "mini-strokes," seldom cause lasting damage. However, they should be taken seriously, and are sometimes called "warning strokes."

Triage Nurse
The first person you'll likely see when you enter the Emergency Room. Determines the severity of each patient's symptoms and the priority in which they will be helped.

Ultrasound
Ultrasound is a test which measures the flow of blood in Arteries. The three main kinds are called B-mode Imaging, Doppler Testing and Duplex Scanning.

Urologist
A bladder and urinary tract doctor.

Vascular
Our system of blood vessels, including Arteries, Veins and Capillaries.

Vein
A blood vessel that carries blood back to the heart.

Vertebral Arteries
Two Arteries that come up from the spinal column to the brain.

Wernicke's Aphasia
People with Wernicke's Aphasia may be able to make

sounds, even words, but have trouble putting them in the right order.

STROKE RESOURCES

Getting Help

For Immediate Help Call 911

Find a Stroke Hospital Near You
The ASA's Interactive Map
http://maps.heart.org/quality/

The NSA's Downloadable List of Hospitals
http://www.stroke.org/site/DocServer/FacilitiesPag
eSCN_2011_4_20.pdf?docID=6741

National Stroke Organizations

The American Stroke Association
http://www.strokeassociation.org

The National Stroke Association
http://www.stroke.org

Understanding Stroke Risk, Warning Signs & Diagnosis

Stroke Risk
http://www.strokeassociation.org/STROKEORG/
AboutStroke/UnderstandingRisk/Understanding-
Risk_UCM_308539_SubHomePage.jsp

Stroke Warning Signs
http://www.strokeassociation.org/STROKEORG/
WarningSigns/Warning-
Signs_UCM_308528_SubHomePage.jsp

Diagnosing Stroke
http://www.strokeassociation.org/STROKEORG/
AboutStroke/Diagnosis/Diagnosis_UCM_310890_A
rticle.jsp

The NSA's Interactive Guide
http://www.stroke.org/site/PageServer?pagename=
explainingstroke

Types of Stroke
http://www.stroke.org/site/PageServer?pagename=t
ype

Stroke Effects
http://www.strokeassociation.org/STROKEORG/
AboutStroke/EffectsofStroke/Effects-of-
Stroke_UCM_308534_SubHomePage.jsp

Patient Education Materials
http://www.strokeassociation.org/STROKEORG/
Professionals/PatientEducationSupport/Patient-
Education-Support_UCM_310901_Article.jsp

Stroke Treatment

From the ASA
www.strokeassociation.org/STROKEORG/AboutSt
roke/Treatment/Treatment_UCM_310892_Article.j
sp

From the NSA
http://www.stroke.org/site/PageServer?pagename=t
reatment

Dealing with the Effects of Stroke

Life After Stroke
http://www.strokeassociation.org/STROKEORG/
LifeAfterStroke/Life-After-
Stroke_UCM_308546_SubHomePage.jsp

Dealing with Paralysis (.pdf)
The NSA's Downloadable Fact Sheet
http://www.stroke.org/site/DocServer/Hemiparesis.
pdf?docID=2803

Dealing with Mobility Issues (.pdf)
The NSA's Downloadable Fact Sheet
http://www.stroke.org/site/DocServer/mobility06.p
df?docID=2801

Dealing with Vision Problems (.pdf)
The NSA's Downloadable Fact Sheet
http://www.stroke.org/site/DocServer/Vision09WE
B.pdf?docID=6821

Dealing with Unpredictable Emotions (.pdf)
The NSA's Downloadable Fact Sheet
http://www.stroke.org/site/DocServer/IEED.pdf?d
ocID=3322

Finding the Right Help After a Stroke

Rehabilitation Hospitals
http://www.stroke.org/site/DocServer/SRNMembe
rsList_0309.pdf?docID=6762

Assisted Living Facilities
http://www.assistedlivingfacilities.org/

Skilled Nursing Facilities
http://www.skillednursingfacilities.org

Home Health Care Agencies
http://www.homehealthcareagencies.com/

http://www.medicare.gov/HomeHealthCompare/

Adult Day Care Services
http://www.helpguide.org/elder/adult_day_care_ce
nters.htm

http://www.eldercare.gov/eldercare.NET/Public/in
dex.aspx

Stroke Support Groups

ADA's Searchable Database of Local Support Groups
http://www.strokeassociation.org/STROKEORG/s
trokegroup/public/zipFinder.jsp

NSA's StrokeSmart Magazine and Searchable Database of Support Groups
http://www.stroke.org/site/PageServer?pagename=
support_groups

Caregiver Support Groups
http://www.strokeassociation.org/STROKEORG/
LifeAfterStroke/ForFamilyCaregivers/For-Family-
Caregivers_UCM_308560_SubHomePage.jsp

Brain and Stroke Images and Illustrations

Downloadable Brochure with Detailed, Full-color Images from the NSA (.pdf).
http://www.stroke.org/site/DocServer/Explaining_
Stroke.pdf?docID=3321

The Same NSA Brochure in Spanish.
http://www.stroke.org/site/DocServer/Explaining_
Stroke_Spanish2.pdf?docID=7163

ASA's Illustrations of the Different Kinds of Strokes
http://www.strokeassociation.org/STROKEORG/
AboutStroke/TypesofStroke/Types-of-
Stroke_UCM_308531_SubHomePage.jsp

ASA's Tour of the Brain
http://www.strokeassociation.org/STROKEORG/
AboutStroke/EffectsofStroke/ATouroftheBrain/A-
Tour-of-the-Brain_UCM_310943_Article.jsp

Downloadable Pamphlets

ASA's List of Patient Information Sheets
http://www.strokeassociation.org/STROKEORG/
AboutStroke/Patient-Information-
Sheets_UCM_310731_Article.jsp

National Stroke Association's Downloadable Brochures
http://www.stroke.org/site/PageServer?pagename=
brochures

NSA's Managing Life Back Home (.pdf)
http://www.stroke.org/site/DocServer/NSAFactShe
et_ManagingLifeatHome.pdf?docID=994

Books, Pamphlets and Videos for Purchase
http://nsa.networkats.com/members_online/membe
rs/createorder.asp

Legal and Financial Assistance

NSA's Medical Benefits and Insurance Fact Sheet (.pdf)
http://www.stroke.org/site/DocServer/NSAFactShe
et_Insurance.pdf?docID=2382

Other Stroke Links

National Association of People with Disabilities
http://www.aapd.com/

Home Health Care Agencies
http://www.homehealthcareagencies.com/
http://www.medicare.gov/HomeHealthCompare/

Adult Day Care Services
http://www.helpguide.org/elder/adult_day_care_ce
nters.htm
http://www.eldercare.gov/eldercare.NET/Public/in
dex.aspx

Assisted Living Facilities
http://www.assistedlivingfacilities.org/

Search for Skilled Nursing Facilities by Zip Code
http://www.skillednursingfacilities.org

ASA's Stroke Connection Magazine and Other Resources
http://www.strokeassociation.org/STROKEORG/
LifeAfterStroke/FindingSupportYouAreNotAlone/Fi
nding-Support-You-Are-Not-
Alone_UCM_308556_SubHomePage.jsp

Visit our website, www.strokebookonline.com
for up-to-the-minute stroke resources.

AUTHORS AND CONTRIBUTORS

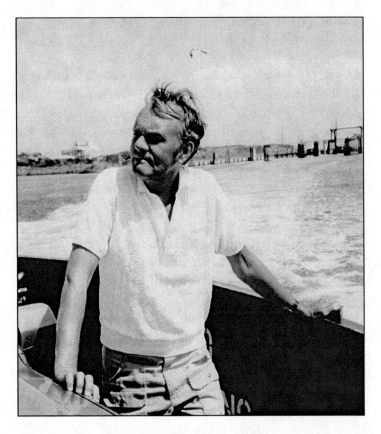

The late **Dr. F. Douglas Prillaman, Ed. D.,** was Professor Emeritus of Special Education at The College of William & Mary in Virginia. He held the Ed.D. from George Washington University, the M.Ed. from William & Mary, and is the principal author of this volume as well as *Diagnostic Prescriptive Teaching*.

Tom Willett, Dr. Prillaman's son, is a former Vice President of Marketing at Sony Entertainment, and the author of more than fifty articles appearing in arts and entertainment magazines.

Dr. S. James Shafer, M.D., Dr. Prillaman's neurologist, is the principal Founder of Vero Neurology. He is Medical Director of the Indian River Medical Center Stroke Center as well as Medical Director of the MS Center of Vero Beach. Dr. Shafer completed his undergraduate work at the University of Florida. He went on to complete medical school and internship at the University of Miami in Florida.

Eleanor W. Prillaman, M. Ed., Dr. Prillaman's wife, holds the B.A. in Sociology from Woman's College of The University of North Carolina and the Masters in Early Childhood Education from Virginia Commonwealth University. She taught at the elementary and junior high school levels, and worked in school social work.

For questions or comments, write
info@strokebookonline.com

For licensing and co-branding inquiries, write
info@alvaaddison.com.

The Road to Recovery

CPSIA information can be obtained at www.ICGtesting.com
Printed in the USA
LVOW13s1711230114

370702LV00001B/151/P